Management and Leadership in Nursing

Management and Leadership in Nursing

Warren F. Stevens, Ph.D.

EXECUTIVE DIRECTOR, AMERICAN ASSOCIATION
OF CRITICAL-CARE NURSES

McGraw-Hill Book Company

NEW YORK   ST. LOUIS   SAN FRANCISCO   AUCKLAND   BOGOTA
DUSSELDORF   JOHANNESBURG   LONDON   MADRID   MEXICO
MONTREAL   NEW DELHI   PANAMA   PARIS   SAO PAULO
SINGAPORE   SYDNEY   TOKYO   TORONTO

MANAGEMENT AND LEADERSHIP IN NURSING

Copyright © 1978 by McGraw-Hill, Inc. All rights reserved. Printed in the United States of America. No part of this publication may be reproduced, stored in a retrieval system, or transmitted, in any form or by any means, electronic, mechanical, photocopying, recording, or otherwise, without the prior written permission of the publisher.

234567890 DODO 7832109

This book was set in Times Roman by Holmes Composition Service. The editor was Orville W. Haberman, Jr.; the designer was Holmes Composition Service; the production supervisor was Jeanne Selzam. The cover was designed by John Hite.
R. R. Donnelley & Sons Company was printer and binder.

Library of Congress Cataloging in Publication Data

Stevens, Warren F
    Management and leadership in nursing.

    Includes index.
    1. Nursing service administration. I. Title.
[DNLM: 1. Leadership. 2. Nursing, Supervisory.
3. Organization and administration. WY105 S846m]
RT89.S75   658'.91'61073   77-8829
ISBN 0-07-061260-9

Contents

v

Part VI

The Future

Preface

The purpose of this book is to address the roles and functions of professional nursing from the point of view of organization and management theory. Many textbooks approach the leadership aspects of nursing without sufficient emphasis on theory of organizations and management. Hence, this book will attempt to fill this gap in the educatory process of nurses by drawing heavily on management functions and organizational structures.

The organization of the book is outlined utilizing a framework familiar to many organization theorists and practicing managers: planning, organizing, directing, and controlling. This approach stresses the systems theory view of management, including the systemic interface problems of subsystems.

Many nurses working in organizations, such as hospitals, outpatient clinics, ambulatory surgical units, and specialized units have asked the question, "I have worked here for years and I know who reports to whom, but why doesn't it work that way on a day-to-day basis?" To address this question, regardless of whether the nurse performs in a staff role, as a team leader, unit director, or director of nursing, this book is written to allow nurses to analyze the formal structure of the organization, the informal structure, and the interfacing of these systems, which results in what they observe and participate in on a daily basis.

This approach will provide a framework of analyzing each management function (planning, organizing, directing, and controlling) in the formal organization followed by the informal or behavioral influences on each function.

Maximum flexibility is possible for the professor who wishes to use various approaches to the delivery of this subject matter. Either the first portion of the course can be structured to approach the formal organization by following the A sections of the book, and then the informal or behavioral influences by using the B sections. If a professor wishes to address each management function from the formal then informal, this can be accomplished by merely sequentially following each chapter.

The author is greatly indebted to Professor Edwin B. Flippo of the University of Arizona for this excellent approach to management and organization theory using a comparative format of formal and informal aspects of these management functions.

To highlight and provide the nurse with an opportunity to apply the concepts developed in each management function, case studies are provided at the conclusion of the book. These case studies will allow the nurse to pretest the acquired knowledge in analyzing management situations prior to using it in a health care setting.

The final chapter looks at the future of organization and management in nursing and examines some theories that espouse the convergence of the formal and informal structures of organizations in nursing.

The author is indebted to many individuals for assistance in preparing this material. Again, Professor Flippo for the approach to this complex subject matter. Professor Jerome P. Lysaught, former Director, National Commission for the Study of Nursing and Nursing Education for his profound insight and knowledge of the problems, opportunities and status of nursing in the United States. For the great input of many colleagues in nursing, members of the Federation of Specialty Nursing Organizations and ANA, Dr. Dorothy Novello, President of NLN, various friends in academia, those administering nursing units and finally, and perhaps most important of all, the bedside nurses throughout the United States for their great input from the firing line.

I am indebted to my wife, Judy Stevens, for enduring the many hours spent during the development of this material and to Ellen French for her accurate and most proficient typing of the manuscript.

Hopefully this book will create a better understanding and practice of management in nursing.

Warren F. Stevens

Management and Leadership in Nursing

Part One

Overview

Part One is designed to demonstrate the great need for knowledge of organization and management theory in nursing. It establishes a background and an understanding of the evolution of various theories of organization.

In Chapter 1 a review of recent developments in health care in general and nursing in particular points to the need for improved organization and management of nursing. The various forces impinging on nursing are examined, including *Abstract for Action,* the federation, professional standards review organizations, and activities of consumer groups.

Chapter 2 provides an evolutionary basis of the development of organization and management theory. Included in this approach are the classical or traditional theory, behavioral theories, management science approaches, and system theory approaches to organizational theory. The development of these approaches will be examined as a foundation for the delivery of concepts throughout the book.

Maximum flexibility is possible for the professor who wishes to use various approaches to this subject matter. The first portion of the course can be structured approach the formal organization by following the A sections of the book and then the informal or behavioral influences by using the B sections. Addressing each management function from the formal then the informal approach can be done by merely following each chapter sequentially. The author is greatly indebted to Professor Edwin B. Flippo of the University of Arizona for this excellent approach to management and organization theory by comparing formal and informal aspects of these management functions.

In addition Chapter 2 looks at the future of organization and management in nursing and examines some theories that espouse the convergence of the formal and informal structures of organizations in nursing.

The author is indebted to many individuals for assistance in preparing this material. Again, Professor Flippo for the approach to this complex subject matter. Professor Jerome P. Lysaught, former Director, National Commission for the Study of Nursing and Nursing Education for his profound insight and knowledge of the problems, opportunities, and status of nursing in the United States. For the great input of many colleagues in nursing, members of the Federation of Specialty Nursing Organizations and ANA, Dr. Dorothy Novello, President of NLN, various friends in academia, those administering nursing units and finally, and perhaps most important of all, the bedside nurses throughout the United States for their great input from the firing line.

I am indebted to my wife, Judy Stevens, for enduring the many hours spent during the development of this material and to Ellen French for her accurate and most proficient typing of the manuscript.

Hopefully this book will bring to bear a better understanding and practice of management in nursing.

Chapter 1

Crisis in Health Care—Need for Organization and Management

During the past decade, the health-care system has been under seige from many individuals and organizations. The attacks have come from outside the direct delivery system and from participants within the system itself. Abraham Ribicoff, U.S. Senator from Connecticut, addressed the status of the health care system in the United States in an article entitled "The 'Healthiest Nation' Myth," which was part of a series called "Health Care R_x for Change" (1970). Numerous other articles have been written about various aspects of the need for change and improvement in the system. Popular magazines have taken up health care as a primary issue, and as a result, the public is reading daily about the many problems inherent in the system that should properly deliver care to patients. Books have been published with such titles as *The Quality of Mercy* (Greenberg, 1971), *The Troubled Calling* (Greenberg, 1968), *Condition Critical: Our Hospital Crisis* (Hoyt, 1966), and *Tender Loving Greed* (Mendelson, 1974). Professional journals have published articles by astute individuals who are familiar with the many problems in health care.

Battistella and Southby (1968) observed that the United States spends more money on health care than does any other country in the world. They cited the problems of maldistribution of physicians and hospital beds. In addition, they noted that:

> There are indications, too, that quality of care has been inferior, especially in terms of antenatal and infant mortality. The whole organisation of medical care in the U.S.A. has failed to respond to changing disease patterns, the move from country to cities, industrialisation, and the increasing proportion of old people in the population. [581]

Dr. Milton Terris (1973, p. 313) observed that "the existence of a crisis in America's health system, declared by the President of the United States in an official statement in July, 1969, has been recognized by an increasingly large section of the population."

These attacks on the general health care delivery system concomitantly have a vital and important implication for nursing.

SYSTEMIC FOCUS—AN EXAMPLE

As the stress level is increasing for improvements in the health care delivery system, nursing must be an integral part of the improvement process. The general system faces problems relating to availability, accessibility, acceptability, comprehensiveness, continuity, quality, and economy. Certainly the health planners, administrators, and institutional boards of directors are principally responsible for the availability of services and their resultant accessibility. The remaining problematical areas of concern are shared among a virtual plethora of health providers in addition to those previously mentioned, namely: physicians, nurses, paramedics, technicians, therapists, social workers, educators, and many more.

The hospital is perhaps one of the most complex organizational forms. The complexity exists regardless of the range or scope of health-care services offered to the patient. Hospitals must continually work to effect the economy of the services rendered to the patients. At all times the quality of care concern must be an overriding issue with economy. Schultz and Johnson (1976, p. 37) describe the systems view of the hospital organization in Figure 1–1. In this approach one might initially assume that nursing is but a small part of the total hospital operation. This certainly is not the case. It has been demonstrated and well documented by many authorities in the field that personnel costs are usually 60 percent to 65 percent of the total operational cost of hospital care and that nursing accounts for the vast majority of those costs to patients.

Nursing will accept responsibility for the quality of nursing care to patients as well as some responsibility for continuity and comprehensive-

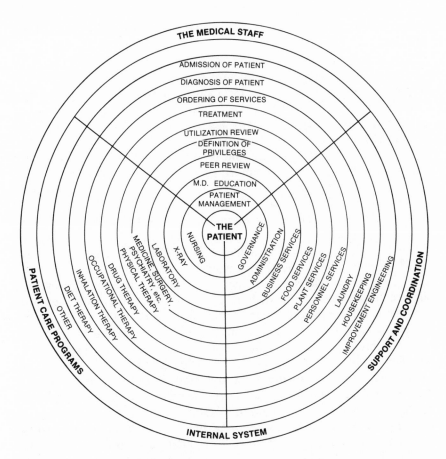

Figure 1-1 Hospital Organization [Reproduced by permission, McGraw-Hill, N.Y., from Shultz & Johnson *Management of Hospitals,* 1976, page 37.]

ness of care. In addition, responsibility is many times assumed for the general acceptability of care. Total responsibility cannot be assumed in some of these areas due to the complexity of care delivered through multicare units and support services. As we are aware, nurses and physicians have not felt the need to address the economy or cost question, since this is the purview and responsibility of the administrator and the board of trustees. Quality and economy are, in fact, the responsibility of all participants in the health care system. If there is to be any hope of addressing these areas of concern, it must come through the development of effective organizational structures that are directed by personnel with management expertise, obtained as an integral part of the educatory process of the health professional, whether it be MD, DO, RN or LPN. This tremendous task cannot be left on the doorstep of the administrator alone.

It must be a team effort by all concerned with the delivery of health care to patients.

In 1973 the federal government passed legislation (Public Law 92-603) to establish professional standards review organizations (PSROS). The purpose of PSROS was to provide mechanisms to review the quality of care delivered to patients including the medical care provided by physicians and the care delivered by nonphysician personnel. The basic thrust of P.L. 92-603 is to address the appropriateness of care delivered and to simultaneously review the care that is to be reimbursed to the citizenry through the various federally funded programs for health care.

Concomitantly with the passage of this law, there was a flurry of activity to establish standards of practice and quality assurance methodologies (Phaneuf, 1972; Zimmer et al., 1974; Ramey, 1973; Wandelt & Phaneuf, 1972; Carter, 1972; Jelinek et al., 1974). Certainly in an area of human life as complex as caring for patients this task is not an easy one. However, these questions relating to standards have never been adequately addressed by practitioners in the health-care setting. Research has been done concerning the nursing process. More recently, research has been directed toward seeking common outcome criteria. The present thinking seems to indicate that an integrated approach, using both process and outcome criteria, is perhaps the most feasible strategy to determine whether or not quality nursing care has been delivered.

Thus, it becomes apparent that the public is asking for more than the assumption of responsibility. It is demanding that health-care providers be fully accountable for delivering care to patients.

In 1969 New York City reported that as consumer representative, government should assess the quality of health services that it purchases from professional and institutional providers of care. Government should be accountable to the taxpayers. Williams (1972, p. 49), a noted authority on responsibility and accountability in health care delivery, shed considerable light on this matter:

> There must be a system for establishing professional standards— standards of behavior, standards of organization, standards for measuring professional practice, etc. There must be a system of surveillance so that you can know if the predetermined standards are being met. There must be a system of enforcement of those standards.

It appears that the health-care system is moving at a very rapid pace through increased responsibility and is facing the day of accountability head on. Are standards of organization and standards for assuring performance at hand to meet these demands? With the increasing pressures on the delivery system to perform, what is the present state of affairs of the profession that delivers a major portion of that care? Can the nursing profession meet this challenge?

CHALLENGE TO NURSING

If a system is to cope with external forces, it must first make an estimate of its own situation. Does nursing possess an inherent cohesiveness that would enable it to present a solid and relatively uniform thrust of resources to meet the many forces impinging on the health care system? This question and others related to the nursing profession were addressed in the report of the National Commission of Nursing and Nursing Education (Lysaught, 1970). The report represented two-and-a-half-years' work examining the status of the nursing profession. Research began by reviewing the early work of Abraham Flexiner's *Medical Education in the United States and Canada* (1960) and Esther Lucile Brown's *Nursing for the Future* (1948). Through its extensive resources, the national commission gained great input into the developments of nursing over time and presented a picture of nursing at the beginning of the 1970s. The commission (Lysaught, 1970), in discussing the problems facing nursing and the trends in nursing, stated, "Nursing stands at a critical point in American history. Because it is an integral part of the entire health industry, nursing is affected by the major movements within our society, in general, and within the health system, in particular." Hence, the great degree of systemic interrelatedness and the nursing interface with the system of health care and society itself became quite clear. Anderson (1968, pp. 31–33) described the forces that act upon nursing in the United States:

> 1　The population will continue to grow in the forseeable future. This will cause both an absolute and a relative increase in those portions of the population that are high users of health service.
> 2　The economy will continue to expand resulting in an increased gross national product and increased discretionary income in both the public and private sectors. Money will be less of a concern though priorities of expenditure will continue to be matters for argument.
> 3　Medical technology will increase in size, complexity, and effectiveness in saving and prolonging life. Many of the people whose lives are extended or saved, however, will require never-ending, closely supervised medical care.
> 4　There will also be an increase in the number of people requiring long-term and basic, custodial care.
> 5　The unit cost of personnel will increase in order to compete with the labor market, and this will intensify the desire for substitutions for registered nurses and will give the registered nurse an increasingly higher status.

6   Associated with this last trend will be an increasing differentiation among registered nurses in clinical specialties.

7   Women of high school age aspiring for professional status will do so through the avenue of the college or university rather than through institutions associated with vocational training.

8   The qualifications for professional attainment will continue to emphasize technical proficiency based on physical and natural sciences rather than nurturance based on behavioral science, feeling, and compassion. This will be one of the problems the nursing profession must watch diligently as it aspires toward higher professional status.

9   The quality and skill of the managers of the health services system will continue to improve. This will result in greater effectiveness, but not necessarily less cost.

Even in the relatively short period of time since the issuance of the commission's study, one can observe that the forces delineated by Anderson are at work. The population continues to grow even though the rate of growth appears to have declined. The median age of the population continues to increase, resulting in a greater proportion of the population demanding health services. Medical technology has provided even greater resources in the care of patients. With the increases in technology, a greater differentiation has occurred within nursing, such that clinical specialization is a reality and is becoming a greater portion of nursing care. As a result of these developments, greater technical proficiency in the physical and natural sciences is being demanded of the professional nurse. The unit cost of personnel has increased as the competing market demands have raised compensation levels. Finally, the quality and skill of the managers of health services have improved through emphasis on short-term seminars to increase managerial expertise.

The area that has received by far the least amount of attention and can have the greatest impact on changes in the system is bringing to bear sufficient organizational structures and management expertise to cause needed changes in the system, as it relates to nursing. The system has tended to promote individuals who possess excellent capabilities in the care of patients to a position where MANAGEMENT OF CARE-GIVING RESOURCES is a principal activity. This change in role has occurred without extensive training for the individual nurse to meet these new and quite different demands.

Lysaught (1975) pointed out the loss of patient contact that occurs with increasing assumption of managerial duties; from staff nurses who spend 50 percent of their time on direct patient care, to the supervisory nurse who spends 17 percent, to the head nurse who spends 7 percent, to finally the director of nursing who has virtually no time in direct patient care. This evolutionary process of moving away from direct patient care has caused many nurses to "want to return to the bedside." The majority of training and education is directed toward patient care and rightly so. However, for those nurses who assume greater managerial responsibility over time, there must be provision in curriculum for management and organization theory, so that the nurse as a manager can be more comfortable and confident in that role.

Douglas and Bevis (1974, p. vii) expressed this problematical situation:

> Education of nurses has traditionally emphasized the study of knowledge and skills of patient care with the assumption that the graduate could function in a leadership role with a minimum of preparation. This preparation was expected to be provided by the employer, who in turn anticipated that the graduate would be able to function in a leadership capacity from the first day of employment with only brief orientation to agency routine and policy. Lack of sufficient leadership preparation has resulted in the nurse's frustration and disenchantment with leadership activities and disillusionment on the part of the employer whose expectations have not been met.

Can the nursing profession meet this need for managerial expertise to provide organizational structures and effective managers to improve nursing care to patients?

The answer must be a resounding *yes*. However, the crucial question must rest in the area of *how* this can become a much needed reality. It must come through a formal preparatory process that is integral to the nursing curriculum. Knowledge of management principles cannot be assumed; it must be acquired through diligent and formal education in the same way that anatomy and physiology are presently incorporated in a nursing course of study.

MANAGEMENT AS A DISCIPLINE IN NURSING

Management is a generic function; it is the organ of leadership, direction, and decision-making in our social institutions. Essentially management faces the same basic tasks in every country and in every society. It must plan and organize work, lead workers toward accomplishment, and obtain desired results. Hence, the manager is responsible for the attainment of those results through tasks, personnel, and physical factors.

It is important to remember that managers *practice* management. Management is a practice and not a science; it can be compared to medicine, law, and engineering.

Drucker (1974, p. 17) delineated the art and practice concepts in contradistinction to science:

Above all, . . . managers practice management. They do not practice economics. They do not practice quantification. They do not practice behavioral science. These are tools for the manager. But he no more practices economics than a physician practices blood testing. He no more practices behavioral sciences than a biologist practices the microscope. He no more practices quantification than a lawyer practices precedents. He practices management.

In the same vein, nursing uses tools as a part of practice: the thermometer, ECG, etc. Those tools alone do not constitute practice, but rather, they assist with tasks to be performed and result in a practice of nursing.

Management has evolved to a point where it is professional in nature. It can be separate and distinct from ownership and rank. Basically, management is an objective function that is predicated on responsibility for effective performance. Hence, nurses as managers are responsible for ensuring that functions are carried out and tasks are performed to meet prescribed plans and objectives of the organization that result in quality patient care. In the near future we will see the emergence of the professional manager in nursing.

MANAGEMENT AND LEADERSHIP

Many writers in nursing have equated the concepts of management and leadership. I contend and will demonstrate throughout this text that leadership is but one part of a much larger concept—that of management. To provide a perspective of leadership as a subsystem of management, a brief explanation of the functions of management will follow. These functions constitute the basis of the development of concepts throughout this text.

Various authorities in the field of management theory have used many terms for the functions of management. In general, the differences of opinion tend to be an emphasis in the use of terms rather than in the content itself.

There is no question that management is getting things done through other people. However, the important point is how the desired results are achieved. They are attained through the functions of management. Thus, we can now define *management* as the planning, organizing, directing, and controlling of operations so that objectives can be achieved effectively.

Flippo (1970, pp. 4–6) defined these functions well:

The first function of the manager is that of PLANNING, that is, the *specification of goals and means*. The resulting plan is composed of goals, policies, procedures, standards and any specification in advance of what is to be done. To implement this plan, an organization must be created. Human and economic resources are divided and allocated to various work areas within the enterprise, and relationships established among the resulting sub-units.

The management function of ORGANIZING is concerned with *developing a structure or framework* which relates all personnel, work assignments and physical resources to each other and to the enterprise objective. This frame-work is usually termed organizational structure.

The third basic management function is that of DIRECTING, which is concerned with *stimulating the organization to undertake action along the lines of the plan.* As such, it deals with the dissemination of orders and the acceptance and execution of these orders. This acceptance and execution usually necessitates managerial attention to training and motivating of individuals and groups that make up the organization. . . .

The final function of management is that of CONTROL, or *regulating whatever . . . action results from direction.* The objective of control is to assure proper performance in accordance with plans. It requires the monitoring of operative performance and the effectiveness of resources utilization. This monitoring provides the management with performance information that can be compared with predetermined plans. In the event of unsatisfactory execution of work, corrective action can take such forms as retraining and remotivating of organization members, altering the allocation of resources through reorganization, and altering the basic plan itself.

Thus, the concept of management encompasses four major functions: planning, organizing, directing, and controlling.

Leadership is a part of the directing function. As we shall see later, directing is the stimulation to undertake action, but concomitantly, the stimulation of the manager is not a necessary and sufficient condition to cause action. The need for acceptance and execution by others is required to obtain the desired results. The understanding of directing as only one of four major functions is essential to effective management. Likewise, the concept of leadership, as a subfunction of directing, is necessary to enable the manager to effectively direct the organization. This important aspect of management will be explained in greater detail later in this book.

SUMMARY

The health-care system has been under attack for the past decade both from inside and outside the system. It was noted that the stress level for improvements in the system is increasing. As an integral and major part of this system, nursing must actively participate in the demanded improvement process. A general review was made of nursing's areas of assumed responsibility. The strong movement from responsibility to accountability in nursing demonstrates the need to tighten the system.

In conjunction with the increased emphasis on accountability, the federal government's role in quality review through PSRO legislation was examined. A flurry of activity has resulted in the areas of standards of practice and quality assurance methodologies. With the pressures of accountability, quality assurance, and economy in nursing, the question was raised as to whether or not the profession was in a position to meet this challenge.

A review of the report of the National Commission on Nursing and Nursing Education and some of its findings regarding trends were explored. Organizational structure and management expertise in nursing are the areas that have received the least amount of emphasis. We cited traditional emphasis in the educatory process of nurses, which stresses the study of knowledge and skills of patient care on the predication that the graduate can function in a leadership role with minimal preparation. The resulting frustration and disillusionment of nurses in this role as well as the lack of meeting employer expectations for leadership was addressed.

A prime contention of this text is that knowledge of management principles cannot be assumed. It must be obtained through diligent and formal education in a similar manner that anatomy and physiology are presently incorporated in a nursing curriculum.

Management was discussed as a discipline in nursing. We noted that it is not a science, but rather a practice in the same sense as medicine, law, or engineering. We examined the professional nature of management, stating that in the near future one can expect to see the professional manager in nursing.

Management and leadership have been equated by many writers in nursing, but leadership is only one part of a much larger concept—management. We defined management as the planning, organizing, directing, and controlling of operations so that objectives can be achieved effectively.

We concluded that leadership is an important part of the directing function, but is not a necessary and sufficient condition to cause action without concomitant acceptance and execution by others to obtain desired results.

BIBLIOGRAPHY

Anderson, O. W. *Toward an Unambiguous Profession? A Review of Nursing.* Chicago: Center for Health Administration Series, Number A6, 1968.

Battistella, Roger M., and Southby, Richard. "Crisis in American Medicine." *Lancet* (March 16, 1968):581–586.

Brown, Esther Lucile. *Nursing for the Future.* New York: Russell Sage Foundation, 1948.

Carter, Joan Haselman et al. *Standards of Nursing Care*. New York: Springer, 1972.

Douglass, Laura Mae, and Bevis, Em Olivia. *Nursing Leadership in Action,* 2nd ed. St. Louis: C. V. Mosby, 1974.

Drucker, Peter F. *Management: Tasks, Responsibilities, and Practices*. New York: Harper & Row, 1973.

Flexner, A. *Medical Education in the United States and Canada*. Boston: D. B. Updike, The Merrymount Press, 1960.

Flippo, Edwin B. *Management: A Behavioral Approach,* 2nd ed. Boston: Allyn & Bacon, 1970.

Greenberg, Selig. *The Troubled Calling*. New York: Atheneum, 1968.

_____. *The Quality of Mercy*. New York: Atheneum, 1971.

Hoyt, Edwin P. *Condition Critical: Our Hospital Crisis*. New York: Holt, Rinehart and Winston, 1966.

Jelinek, R. C. et al. *A Methodology for Monitoring Quality of Nursing Care*. Washington D.C.: U.S. Government Printing Office, Department of Health, Education, and Welfare Publication (HRA) No. 74–25, January 1974.

Lysaught, Jerome P. *An Abstract for Action*. New York: McGraw-Hill, 1970.

_____. "Keynote Speech", American Association of Critical-Care Nurses' Second National Teaching Institute, Boston, Mass., May 1975.

MacEachern, Malcolm T. *Hospital Organization and Management*. Berwyn, Ill. Physicians' Record, 1962.

McCleery, Robert. *One Life—One Physician*. Washington D.C.: Public Affairs Press, 1971.

Mendelson, Mary A. *Tender Loving Greed*. New York: Knopf, 1974.

Phaneuf, Maria C. *The Nursing Audit: Profile for Excellence*. New York: Appleton-Century-Crofts, 1972.

Ramey, Irene G. "Setting Nursing Standards and Evaluating Care." *Journal of Nursing Administration* (May–June 1973): 27–35.

Ribicoff, Abraham. "The 'Healthiest Nation' Myth, Health Care: R_x for Change." *Saturday Review* (August 22, 1970): 18–20.

Terris, Milton. "Crisis and Change in America's Health System." *American Journal of Public Health* 63: 313–318.

Wandelt, Mabel A., and Phaneuf, Maria C. "Three Instruments for Measuring the Quality of Nursing Care." *Hospital Topics* (August 1972): 21–29.

Williams, K. J. "Beyond Responsibility: Toward Accountability." *Hospital Progress* (January 1972): 44–50.

Zimmer, M. J.; Lang, N. M.; and Miller, D. J. *Development of Sets of Patient Health Outcome Criteria by Panels of Nurse Experts*. Madison, Wisc.: Wisconsin Regional Medical Program, 1974.

Chapter 2

Evolution of Organization and Management Theory

Today, nurse-managers operate in an environment that is in a state of continuous flux. Managers must be thoroughly familiar with a plurality of factors that influence the conditions under which care-giving resources are managed. It is imperative that the most current information be available, since information is important to the understanding of facts. For nurse-managers, facts generally imply problems, and problems require solutions.

What approaches are available to managers for securing solutions to problems in the execution of the decision-making process? Certainly, managers use different approaches in the interpretation, analysis, and solution of nursing management problems. In many cases, the complexity of the problem provides an indication of the most appropriate method of analysis. Through experience and knowledge, nurses can scan the problem and secure a preliminary decision that could be appropriate, but at other times, such a decision might not be sufficient for finding a solution.

Managerial approaches to problem solving may be classified into various categories. For purposes of this discussion, the approaches are categorized as follows: historical, parasitic, and professional.

The historical approach is used by the managers who, in addressing problems, follow the same processes and techniques that were handed down from the past. These managers lack innovative ideas. They base their solutions on the repetition of previous approaches to previous problems. The prevailing hope of the historical manager is that the present problem is sufficiently similar to the past problem that the old solution will be relevant to the new problem. Historical managers expend much energy in attempting to "force fit" the new problem into an old solution. Of course, this approach does not consider the extent of the changes occurring in the new environment, either internal or external. The degree of this changing environment was well described by Alvin Toffler in *Future Shock* (1970). As a result, this approach is in contradistinction to the prevailing dynamism so evident in the nurse-manager's working environment.

The parasitic approach consists of observing and learning from the actions of other managers. This approach differs from the historical one in that managers attempt to copy the behavior and actions of colleagues rather than duplicating the methods of a predecessor. Although some improvement in managerial decision making can be learned from this approach, it still presents the problem of fitting the solution to the right problem.

Professional managers are characterized by the use of theoretical systems in search of solutions to problems. As members of a profession, these managers are subject to the common characteristics of a profession: "level of commitment, disciplined educational process, unique body of knowledge and skill, active and cohesive professional organization; and discretionary authority and judgement" (Lysaught, 1970, p. 32). This book will attempt to provide some of the foundation necessary to your becoming a professional manager. Certainly, the level of commitment must come from individuals engaging in the active pursuit of their occupation throughout the productive years of their lives. As students of management you are presently engaged in a disciplined educational process, and hopefully this material will help provide part of the unique body of knowledge and skill you need as effective managers. The active and cohesive professional organization is available, and through the execution of your responsibilities as nurse-managers, you will have discretionary authority and judgement.

Throughout the sections of this book, you will be provided with an interdisciplinary approach using a systems model, which will provide you with a theoretical framework for the solution of problems. Practical experience gained throughout your career will build and reinforce your decision-making powers based on the theoretical framework.

The pretension of restricting actual nursing problems to fixed solutions is not logical and is, at best, erroneous. Such restrictions on nurse-managers result in ineptness and are evidenced by the *Peter Principle* in action. To preclude such ineptness, it is imperative that the students of management be presented the various schools of management as such schools evolved over time. Exposure to the pioneer thinkers on management is essential. The theories and practices that were initially developed are continually referred to in the literature, and the concepts are used today in the practice of management.

The schools of management to be examined will be the traditional, behavioral, and management science. You should realize from the outset that each has some limitations. Consequently, effective nurse-managers should use them in an eclectic way.

TRADITIONAL SCHOOL

American engineer Frederick Winslow Taylor is considered the founder of the traditional school. He began his career in the 1870's in a small machine shop in Philadelphia. After working as an apprentice, he became a machinist foreman. While in this position, he began work that would make him famous as "the father of scientific management."

Taylor stated his concept as "knowing exactly what you want men to do, and then seeing that they do it in the best and cheapest way" (Taylor, 1910, p. 21). Taylor's essential thesis is that management can be considered a process using the scientific method. Most of Taylor's work was managing production in a factory. The primary problem he addressed was "how much work was it reasonable to expect from an individual for a given job." At that time estimates had been obtained principally from observation or by actually performing the job. Attempting to secure a standard for a job resulted in much argument. Therefore, Taylor obtained the services of an individual to time each motion with a stopwatch. Jobs were subdivided into elements, and each element was timed, resulting in the development of a standard. Taylor's work represents one of the beginnings of time-and-motion study. Shortly thereafter, industry began using this approach on a systematic basis.

Through Taylor's efforts, management began studying all aspects of its operations scientifically and developed standards that were predicated on a logical, rational, and consistent basis. Taylor's approach to organization was characterized by specialization, division of labor, sequence of work, planning and evaluation of equipment, and all interrelated functions. Under Taylor's differential work plan, an individual could increase earnings by increasing production. However, those individuals who had not met the standards suffered greatly because substandard production rates were depressed to allow for the high rates used for high production. In many cases "unfair situations" developed. Taylor's approach gave insufficient consideration to bottlenecks in the assembly line or malfunctioning equipment.

These problems were somewhat alleviated by Henry Lawrence Gantt, an associate of Taylor's. Gantt developed an incentive plan based on the production of a number of pieces in a day. Workers received a daily wage regardless of completing their daily quota, but they also received extra pay for work above the quota. This approach established standard hours measured in terms of work, so that an individual who completed twelve standard hours of work in eight hours would be paid for twelve hours. Thus, Taylor showed the method, and its application was demonstrated by Gantt. To provide a mechanism for comparison of actual production performance with established standards, Gantt developed charts to permit such comparisons. Work planned and work performed were illustrated on the same chart with reference dates for scheduling, dispatching, and control.

Contemporaries of Taylor and Gantt, Frank and Lillian Gilbreth devoted their efforts to motion analysis "to find and perpetuate the scheme of least-waste method of labor" (Gilbreth, 1912). Their approach focused not on how long it took to do a piece of work but, rather, on the best way to do it. Under Gilbreth's definition, the "one best way" was the one that required the fewest motions to accomplish. This complementary work to Taylor's time study was a major contribution to the field of motion analysis.

Although Taylor, Gantt, and the Gilbreths focused on the techniques that management might use on the production of goods, none of them addressed management as a function distinct and separate from the techniques.

Henri Fayol made an attempt to develop a broad and more universal approach to management. Fayol was a French-born engineer who was chief executive of a coal and steel combine for 30 years. In 1916 he published a study concerned with the principles of general management entitled *General and Industrial Management*. Fayol's work provided definitions regarding the basic functions for management. He came to the conclusion that there was a set of management principles that could be used in all types of management situations regardless of the organization. Fayol's use of the term *principle* was only for convenience; they were intended as guides and not as immutable laws. His book is now considered a classic in management literature and is the forerunner of modern textbooks that deal with the principles of management. Fayol's basic functions of management are planning, organizing, commanding, coordinating, and controlling (Fayol, 1949). He primarily studied the upper echelon of the organization. Fayol noted that the principles of management are flexible (not absolute) and should be used according to specific conditions and situations.

The overall approach of Taylor, Gantt, the Gilbreths, and Fayol was to provide a rational basis for management and place it on a more objective and scientific foundation. Their work has done much to increase the productivity of the United States and the world. Modern management still uses these traditional concepts as a basis for management in the United States.

Harold Koontz (1961) has summarized the fundamental beliefs of the traditional school of management theory as follows:

1 That managing is a process and can best be dissected intellectually by analyzing the functions of the manager

2 That long experience with management in a variety of enterprise situations can be grounds for distillation of certain fundamental truths or generalizations—usually referred to as principles—which have a clarifying and predictive value in the understanding and improvement of managing

3 That these fundamentals can become focal points for useful research both to ascertain their validity and to improve their meaning and applicability in practice

4 That such truths can furnish elements, at least until disproved, and certainly until sharpened, of a useful theory of management

5 That managing is an art, but one like medicine and engineering, which can be improved by reliance on the light and understanding of principles

6 That the principles in management, like principles in the biological and physical sciences, are nonetheless true even if a prescribed treatment or design by a practitioner in a given case situation chooses to ignore a principle and the costs involved, or attempts to do something else to offset the costs incurred (this is, of course, not new in medicine, engineering, or any other art, for art is the creative task of compromising fundamentals to attain a desired result)

7 That, while the totality of culture and of the physical and biological universe has varying effects on the manager's environment and subjects, as indeed it does in every other field of science or art, the theory of management does not need to encompass the field of all knowledge in order for it to serve as a scientific or theoretical foundation.

Thus, the general approach of the traditional school is to examine the functions of managers. Many academicians and practitioners have given considerable thought to the dissection and analysis of the concepts and functions of this school. The result has been a refinement of the traditional school.

BEHAVIORAL SCHOOL

As more managers began operating under the principles of the traditional school of management thought, it became apparent that results were not totally compatible with prior expectation. Many managers felt that the traditional approach did not possess sufficient concepts to provide a complete theory of management. Much of this thinking evolved from the work and writings of Elton Mayo (1933) and F. J. Roethlisberger (1939). They observed that the manager operating under the fundamental principles of the traditional school were not necessarily the most efficient. In addition, the management systems did not always work as conceived. What factor or factors could create this seeming incongruence of the a priori expectations and the pragmatic realities of real life situation results?

An attempt to validate the generally accepted principles of management by Mayo and Roethlisberger resulted in a major conclusion concerning the traditional school; specifically, it had generally not considered the human aspect of organizations. This provided the basis for a new school of thought in management. Initially called the human relations movement, it later became known as the behavioral school.

It is interesting to examine briefly the research that led to these most important findings. In the 1920s Mayo had joined a group that was researching a premise of the Gilbreths regarding worker fatigue and productivity. The research conducted at the Hawthorne plant of Western Electric in Chicago attempted to validate the following results of the fatigue study (Spriegel & Myers, 1953, p. 309)—"that more output can be achieved by applying oneself for short periods, and then resting, than by applying oneself less steadily and having no rest periods."

The research of the Hawthorne experiments was expected to show that under controlled conditions the manipulation of a single variable (namely, the rest period) would validate the Gilbreth premise. The general expectation that introducing rest periods or breaks would result in increased productivity was initially observed. However, when the rest periods were removed from the work schedule, the researchers noted that productivity was at a higher level than before the commencement of the experiment (a time when no rest periods had been allowed). Rest periods were reintroduced with an even higher level of productivity. After several years of the Hawthorne experiment (from 1927 to 1932), there was a noted increase in productivity over time, which demonstrated that the rest period variable possessed an independent character relative to productivity. Thus, "other factors" must have accounted for the productivity increase in this "controlled experiment." The conclusion indicated that the human factor had not been controlled.

In the development of the behavioral school, Chester Barnard is recognized as one of the outstanding contributors to the behavioral movement. In 1938 Barnard who had served as president of the New Jersey Bell Telephone Company wrote *The Functions of the Executive*. This work was primarily drawn from sociological approaches to management in which Barnard attempted to find answers underlying the process of management. Barnard established a theory for a system of cooperation. This theory basically emphasized the need of individuals to solve the limitation of themselves and their environment through cooperation with others. Barnard's work brought forth the recognition of the organization as a social organism that must interact with environmental pressures and conflict. *The Functions of the Executive* expanded the scope of understanding in management by adding sociological aspects to management.

According to Tannenbaum, Wechsler, and Massarik (1961, p. 9), the behavioral school as it has evolved over time brings to bear "existing and newly developed theories, methods, and techniques of the relevant social sciences upon the study of inter- and intrapersonal phenomena, ranging from the personality dynamics of individuals at one extreme to the relation of cultures at the other."

The primary stress of the behavioral school is the consideration of the organization as groups of individuals working to accomplish objectives. Some proponents of this school view it from the perspective of a total management approach, whereas others view it as a necessary partner with the traditional school to enhance the overall effectiveness of the organization. However, as the traditional school stood alone and was incomplete, so the behavioral school is likewise incomplete if it were to stand alone.

MANAGEMENT SCIENCE SCHOOL

The final management school is that of management science. For purposes of this discussion, the areas of decision making and quantitative methods will be considered in this school.

Decision making concentrates on a rational approach to making a decision. The decision becomes the central focus of all management, implying thorough consideration of alternatives prior to the selection of a course of action. This basis of thinking is an outgrowth of the field of economics. The areas of concern include indifference curves, marginal costs-benefits and utility, problems of maximization, decisions under partial information, use of nonparametric methods of analysis, and so on. The approach has been heavily grounded in the use of quantitative methods. Thus, the management science school views management as a system of mathematical models and processes. Solutions to management problems are obtained through the use of techniques such as simulation, linear regression, quadratic programming, input-output analysis, and queueing theory. Individuals working in these areas are commonly referred to as operations researchers, operation analysts, and systems engineers.

The management science school has brought the view of decision theory and mathematical models to modern management. As a result, a more definitive approach to the formulation of problems and solutions has come to pass. According to Koontz (1961, pp. 181–182), the usefulness of mathematical approaches to any field of interest, "forces upon the researcher the definition of a problem or problem area it conveniently allows the insertion of symbols for unknown data, and its logical methodology, developed by years of scientific application and abstraction, furnishes a powerful tool for solving or simplifying complex phenomena."

Certainly the decision theory and mathematical model concepts of the management science school are most helpful to management as tools. But decision-making is a portion of what management does and is not management itself, regardless of the entire organization. In a similar sense, mathematical modeling of problems is not management of the organization, but rather methods that provide management with greater powers for analysis of problems. Consequently, the management science view represents tools that managers can use to assist them in the practice of management and cannot by itself be management.

SUMMARY

Nurse-managers operate in a dynamic environment that places heavy demands on them to cope with a plurality of factors influencing the conditions under which care-giving resources are managed. Managerial approaches to decision making were defined as historical, parasitic, and professional. We observed that the historical and parasitic approaches contradicted the prevailing dynamism so evident in the working nurse-managers' environment. Professional nurse-managers were characterized as those who use theoretical systems in search of problems and solutions to problems.

We examined the schools of management to provide a background of management thought, and we noted that each school has some limitations. Consequently, effective nurse-managers should use them in an eclectic manner.

The traditional school was reviewed, covering the work of pioneers such as Taylor, Gantt, the Gilbreths, and Fayol. This school provided a more rational basis for management and placed it on a more objective and scientific foundation. Concepts of time-and-motion study, one best way, and the functions of general management as brought forth by these pioneer leaders were reviewed.

The establishment of the behavioral school was examined through the work of Mayo and Roethlisberger during the Hawthorne experiments. These experiments, which were intended to validate some premises of the Gilbreths, provided insight into the great need for consideration of the human aspects of management. The work of Chester Barnard as published in *The Functions of the Executive* added a sociological dimension to management practice and helped increase the understanding of the practice of management.

The final management school of thought—namely, the management science school—was reviewed. This school combines decision theory and quantitative methods. Decision theory is primarily an outgrowth of economics. Both areas are thought to enhance the effectiveness of management through the use of logical methodologies, which provided powerful tools for solving complex phenomena. However, we noted that the management science view represents tools that managers can use to improve effectiveness, but it does not constitute total management.

BIBLIOGRAPHY

Barnard, Chester I. *The Functions of the Executive*. Cambridge, Mass.: Harvard University Press, 1930.

Fayol, Henri. *General and Industrial Management*. New York: Pitman, 1949 (translated from the French originally published in 1916).

Gilbreth, F. B. *Primer of Scientific Management*, Princeton, N.J.: D. Van Nostrand, 1912.

Koontz, Harold. "The Management Theory Jungle." *Journal of the Academy of Management*, vol. 4, no. 3 (December 1961): 174–188.

Lysaught, Jerome P. *An Abstract for Action*. New York: McGraw-Hill, 1970.

Mayo, Elton. *The Human Problems of an Industrial Civilization*, Cambridge, Mass.: Harvard University Press, 1933.

Roethlisberger, F. J., and Dickson, William J. *Management and the Worker*. Cambridge, Mass.: Harvard University Press, 1939.

Spriegel, William R., and Myers, Clark E., eds. *The Writings of the Gilbreths*. Homewood, Ill.: Richard D. Irwin, 1953.

Tannenbaum, Robert; Wechsler, I. R.; and Massarik, Fred. *Leadership and Organization: A Behavioral Science Approach*. New York: McGraw-Hill, 1961.

Taylor, F. W. *Shop Management*. New York: Harper, 1910.

Toffler, Alvin. *Future Shock*. New York: Bantam Books, 1970.

Part Two

Organizational Planning in Nursing

Part Two contains concepts in formal organizational planning that examine the development of organizational goals and objectives (Section A). In addition, the behavioral influences on planning are considered, including the needs of the individual nurse and integration of the nurse into the organizational milieu (Section B).

Chapter 3 reviews planning concepts, including goals, objectives, policies, and procedures. The interrelationship and complementary nature of these concepts are examined from various levels of definitization.

Chapter 4 provides the foundation for the development of formal organizational plans. Strategic and tactical planning concepts are discussed, including the basic components of plans: ends, means, resources, implementation, and control. Detail planning, including nursing care planning, is reviewed.

Chapter 5 examines the needs of individual nurses, including Maslow's hierarchy of needs as well as the concepts of self, personality, and maturation. The basic nature of individuals as viewed by McGregor through Theory X and Theory Y is reviewed.

Chapter 6 examines the nurse/organizational interface. A new employee situation is used to demonstrate the expectations of individual nurses, including compensation, job security, association, acceptance, and recognition. Organizational adaptation and employee motivation concepts are covered. In addition, the concepts of individual differences, individual adaptation, and external job factors are considered at length.

Chapter 3

Organizational Goals and Objectives

The vast majority of nurse-managers practice in a hospital setting. In order to operate as effective managers in a health care institution, it is imperative that they understand the purpose, goals, and objectives of the organization.

Certainly the general overriding purpose of the hospital as an organization is to render care to the sick and injured. The essential focus then stresses what the organization is trying to accomplish. However, a greater refinement of even the general direction of the organization is needed if one is to ascertain a better understanding of "what" the organization is trying to do. In addition, some mechanism is essential to provide benchmarks by which progress can be measured. There must be an evaluation process to indicate "how" the organization is doing.

PLANNING TERMINOLOGY

Before delving into an extensive and complex discussion of goals, objectives, programs, tasks, activities, etc., it is necessary to define the terms.

Organizations are developed to fill a need or address a problem of some type. From a definitive statement of a need or problem, a mission is

25

perceived and goals identified. A problem statement is *the identification of existing or anticipated conditions or obstacles that must be removed or ameliorated to enable the achievement of a goal.* A goal is *a statement identifying a perceived mission or responsibility for which programs are planned. A goal should be broad but realistic, specify no definite time for accomplishment, not be quantitative, and not indicate a specific output to be measured.*

Once the problem statement has been secured and the formulation of goals obtained, it is imperative that more definitive thinking be applied to determine a measurable phenomenon that can be accomplished in a particular time frame. To reach this level of refinement, organizational objectives are necessary. Objectives are *statements of a condition or of a specific result desired within an identified period of time for accomplishing a goal.* Thus, we see a progressive refinement from the problem statement to the establishment of goals to their subsequent definition as measurable objectives.

GOALS

Management is constantly bombarded by articles on "how to set organizational goals." Many articles have stressed the appropriateness of one goal over another. It must be realized from the outset that organizations do not have just one goal, but rather a multitude of goals. To properly approach the establishment of goals, it is essential that a conceptual framework be developed that will embrace the whole range of goals in order to use them and their subsequent objectives in an efficient manner.

As we mentioned in the discussion of managerial approaches to problem solving (i.e., historical, parasitic, and professional), management practice in nursing alone cannot provide sufficient armament for the many problems that face nurse-managers today.

This condition is even further exacerbated in the development of goals and objectives. Lyndall Urwick (1952) described this situation well:

> We cannot do without theory. It will always defeat practice in the end for a quite simple reason. Practice is static. It does and does well what it knows. It has, however, no principle for dealing with what it doesn't know. . . . Practice is not well adapted for rapid adjustment to a changing environment. Theory is light-footed. It can adapt itself to changed circumstances, think out fresh combinations and possibilities, peer into the future. (p. 10)

Thus, the goals of the organization, whether implicit or explicit, provide the direction that will lend unity and continuity to a variety of tasks and activities as it moves toward the future.

Philip Selznick (1957, p. 144) has stated that, "Goal setting, if it is to be institutionally meaningful, is framed in the language of character or identity; that is, it tells us what we should do in order to become what we want to be."

Goals are usually stated in terms of values and public services to be rendered to either meet a perceived need and/or alleviate a problem (Donabedian, 1973, p. 1), so it would not be unusual for an organization such as a hospital to state goals as follows:

1. The purpose and responsibility of the hospital is to render care to the sick and injured.

2. The delivery of health care in the hospital will reflect the fact that it is a privilege and responsibility to care for the sick with respect and compassion at all times.

3. The client (or patient) is a guest in the house and is to be considered the most important person in the hospital.

4. The recovery and restoration to health of the client (or patient) is of utmost importance to our being and existence.

5. The hospital shall provide quality health care to all clients (or patients).

6. The hospital shall attempt to effect cost containment with regard to the delivery of health services.

The general goals as stated are somewhat changed from the recent past which demonstrates that goals are dynamic and will change over time. As the goals collectively express the mission of the organization, it must be realized that the mission has dynamic characteristics. According to Drucker (1973, p. 89), "very few definitions of the purpose and mission of a business have any life expectancy of thirty, let alone fifty, years. To be good for ten years is probably all one can normally expect." For this reason, many hospitals have updated and revised their goals in recent years to reflect the increased emphasis on quality of care review. Many state and federal government agencies have also been placing considerable pressure on the hospitals to demonstrate greater control of costs.

In each organizational setting there exists a hierarchical structure of organizational goals that are interrelated and are generally mutually supportive.

In most hospital organizations, nursing is an operational department; they will usually establish an overall philosophy that is supportive of the mission of the total organization. Such a philosophy will refer to the value of the individual, to the acceptance of responsibility for providing optimal nursing care to clients and the provision of a conducive environment for client recovery and development of each health care provider.

Goals developed from these philosophical statements produce a greater refinement and elaboration of the philosophy. Moss and others (1966, p. 261) illustrate through their research a typical example of the goals of a nursing department:

1   To provide individualized nursing care for each patient considering his emotional, spiritual, mental, physical, social and health education needs.

2   To keep the nurse patient-centered in his/her thinking, though he/she accepts additional responsibilities as a result of expanding health programs.

3   To cooperate with the medical profession and other health fields to the achievement of total health care of the patient.

4   To cooperate with hospital administration and other hospital services to provide facilities and an environment conducive to optimum care of the patient.

5   To improve the quality of nursing care by good administration, supervision, teaching and effective evaluation of all nursing personnel.

6   To maintain an environment that will develop the understanding and skills of each member of the nursing team and promote job satisfaction.

7   To conduct and participate in research which is directed toward better care of all patients.

8   To interpret nursing to the community.

9   To provide clinical areas for student nurses in the educational programs.

It must be realized that organizations are complex things. Every individual member has his or her own values, aspirations, and goals. (These aspects of individuals will be covered in Chapter 5 and 6). Goals must be viewed as dynamic; they cannot fit into a world of constancy. There must be a continual reevaluation of or reappraisal of goals. Thompson and McEwen (1958) stress the importance of the fact that organizations must reappraise their goals on a continuing basis in light of changing needs and demands. The more frequently this reappraisal occurs, the more likely the organization is to adapt to and meet the changing needs of the environment. This situation represents an ongoing process that should be accomplished at least annually to ensure relevancy of the organization to its environment.

Many times a problem arises between what is known as the stated goal and the real goal. Etzioni (1964) and Perrow (1961) have done a lot of research and analysis on this most important concept. The general tendency is for organizational operants to deviate from the stated goals as delineated in the articles of incorporation and official positions of the organization. This divergence or disparity is commonly referred to as "goal displacement." The obvious implication is that the initially defined goals in a legitimate sense are somewhat less served by the organizational participants.

POLICY

The linking factor that ties goals to objectives is known as policy. Policy is normally and best set by a board of directors (or board of trustees). As the goals are subdivided and explicitly stated in terms of quantifiable results in a discrete time frame, the policies as promulgated by the board provide general guidance and direction for the accomplishment of goals. Therefore, we shall define policy as *a general guideline established on a predetermined basis to provide direction for the organization, ensuring future action.*

Thus, we see the goals of the organization as statements for the accomplishment of ends, interfaced and coupled with policy positions that provide a direction for accomplishing the goal as stated. The policy direction is the basis for procedures that will follow as implementation strategies for objectives of the organization.

Objectives as previously stated refer to a statement, condition, or specific result desired within an identified period of time for accomplishing a goal. Objectives are not normally developed for the overall organization, but rather apply to the divisions and departments of the organization in meeting overall organizational goals.

A nursing department may delineate the objectives for a particular operating year as follows:

1. To increase the accuracy of nursing diagnosis by 10 percent over the previous year in the department within the next calendar year.
2. To decrease hospitalization of clients by an amount of one-half day given a relatively constant patient mix as compared to the prior years' experience and without resulting in necessary readmission within the next calendar year.
3. To reduce registered nursing staff requirements by 10 percent by using less-trained personnel for more routine duties of registered nurses within the next calendar year.
4. To provide a 20 percent increase in community programs for interpreting the role of nursing to the community within the next calendar year.
5. To improve the quality of nursing care delivered within the next calendar year by reducing the number of client cases regarded as exceptions by 10 percent for review by the committee on quality review.
6. To increase the number of continuing education offerings to professional staff by 15 percent over the amount offered in the previous calendar year.

7. To reduce professional staff turnover by 10 percent from the previous year by enhancing the environment for delivery of care to clients.

The problem of stated versus real objectives usually develops as it does with goals. However, the divergence is generally less than with goals, due to objectives' more specific definitions.

As goals must be viewed in a dynamic sense, so must objectives. The degree of objectives' dynamism is certainly more exacerbated because of their relative shorter time frame. Since objectives are usually stated for a one- to five-year time period and since goals are defined for a five- to ten-year period, the review and reappraisal of objectives must be accomplished more often and in many cases is done on a continuous basis. It can be reasoned that if objectives deviated significantly from their originally intended end result, then there seems to be little hope that the goal that the objective supports can be achieved. Thus, it becomes imperative that the relevancy of the objectives of the department or organizational subunit be constantly reviewed.

PROCEDURE

As the linking factor of the goal to the objective was the policy, so the linking factor of the objective to the position description is the procedure. Generally the procedure is developed by the department head or the supervisor as a mechanism to accomplish the objective as stated. The procedure then delineates the specifics required to accomplish the objectives; it tells how the objective will be met on a step-by-step basis. Therefore, we shall define procedure as *a series of functions established on a predetermined basis to provide for the accomplishment of a specific endeavor.*

The objectives of the department or organizational subunit represent a statement of accomplishment of specific end results and is interfaced with procedures to provide a direction for the accomplishment of objectives as stated. The procedures as developed provide a basis for the establishment of staffing positions. This matter will be covered in later chapters.

Once the goals, policies, objectives, and procedures have been established, we can discuss the plans of the organization, which is the subject of our next chapter.

SUMMARY

In order to operate in an effective manner, nurse-managers must understand the purpose, goals, and objectives of the organization. From the establishment of an organization, some overriding purpose should be stated and delineated. Once this has been accomplished, the organization must establish some long-range goals to meet its intended purpose. A goal was defined as a statement identifying a perceived mission or responsibility for which programs are planned. A goal should be broad and realistic, specify no definite time for accomplishment; it should not be qualitative, and it should not indicate a specific output to be measured. We noted that organizations do not have just one goal, but, rather, have a multitude of goals. Goals are normally stated in terms of values and public services to be rendered to meet either perceived needs and/or alleviate a problem. The dynamic nature of goals was stated and recognized.

The linking factor of goals to objectives is known as policy and provides a general guideline of direction for the organization to ensure future action. Policy is normally established by a board of directors.

Once goals are determined, organizations further define goals into operational objectives that represent a statement, condition, or specific result desired within an identified period of time. It was noted that objectives are usually established for a department or organizational subunit. Once objectives have been determined, procedures are written to assist in the implementation of the objectives. Procedures are a series of functions established on a predetermined basis to provide for the accomplishment of a specific endeavor. Collectively the goals, policies, objectives, and procedures provide the foundation for various levels of organizational plans.

BIBLIOGRAPHY

Ackoff, Russell L. *A Concept of Corporate Planning*. New York: Wiley-Interscience, 1970.

Donabedian, Avedis. *Aspects of Medical Care Administration: Specifying Requirements for Health Care*. Cambridge, Mass. Harvard University Press, 1973.

Drucker, Peter F. *Management: Tasks, Responsibilities, Practices*. New York: Harper & Row, 1973.

Etzioni, A. *Modern Organizations*. Englewood Cliffs, N.J.: Prentice-Hall, 1964.

Jenkins, A. L., ed. *Emergency Department Organization and Management*. St. Louis: C. V. Mosby, 1975.

Koontz, Harold, and O'Donnell, Cyril. *Management: A Book of Readings*. New York: McGraw-Hill, 1972.

Mali, Paul. *Managing by Objectives*. New York: Wiley-Interscience, 1972.

Moss, Arthur B. et al. *Hospital Policy Decisions: Process and Action*. New York: Putnam's Sons, 1966.

Odiorne, George S. *Management by Objectives: A System of Managerial Leadership*. New York: Pitman, 1965.

Perrow, C. "The Analysis of Goals in Complex Organizations." *American Sociological Review* 26 (December 1961): 854–866.

Schulz, Rockwell, and Johnson, Alton C. *Management of Hospitals*. New York: McGraw-Hill, 1976.

Selznick, Philip. *Leadership in Administration*. Evanston, Ill.: Row-Peterson, 1957.

Thompson, J. D., and McEwen, W. J. "Organizational Goals and Environment: Goal-Setting as an Interaction Process." *American Sociological Review* 23 (February 1958): 23–31.

Urwick, Lyndall. "Notes on the Theory of Organization." New York: American Management Association, 1952.

Chapter 4

Formal Organizational Plans

Formal plans of organizations are attempts to anticipate a future desired result and to take the necessary steps to cause them to happen. Ackoff (1970, p. 1), a well-known consultant and teacher has described the nature of planning, "Wisdom is the ability to see the long-run consequences of current actions, the willingness to sacrifice short-run gains for larger long-run benefits, and the ability to control what is controllable and not to fret over what is not. Therefore, the essence of wisdom is concern with the future. It is not the type of concern with the future that the fortune teller has; he only tries to predict it. The wise man tries to control it."

Planning is the specification in advance of goals and means, where means includes planning for resourceful implementation strategies and control mechanisms (Flippo, 1970, p. 4).

At the outset of this discussion on planning, it is absolutely essential that a "feeling" be developed about the nature of planning itself. Planning consists of two properties both of which are necessary to obtain desired future results. The end product of these efforts is a written plan. Many individuals falsely believe that once a plan has been developed and published it is, in fact, "carved in stone." This is definitely not the case. The written plan represents only an interim report in the planning process. Therefore, planning is not simply an act at a point in time, but rather an ongoing process that does not have a final conclusion or finite end point. As a process, it permits iteration toward a solution to problems, but it never reaches a complete finality as many individuals often suspect (Sayles & Chandler, 1971, p. 61). When a decision is made, a commitment of resources to projects occurs. However, in the purest sense of the word, the decision predicated on the plan and other information is, at best, based on partial or incomplete information at that time. Hence, nurses operating in the decision-making role must make the decision under conditions of risk and uncertainty. The reason for the iteration toward a solution versus finality of the decision stems from the very nature of the planning process. There is no specific limitation on the number of times that the decision maker can review action taken in the past. In addition, the actual operating organization and its operating environment are in a dynamic state; consequently, these decisions are limited by the concept of bounded rationality. This concept, coined by Herbert Simon, reflects the fact that decisions must be made within the confines of our knowledge and information level at the time they are made. It is reasoned that the decision maker cannot take all possible changes occurring within the organization or its environment into account at the time of the decision.

It must be realized by nurse decision makers that planning is a continuous process that is under constant revision and reevaluation. This dynamic nature of planning is essential to ensure the relevancy of the plan and its resultant decisions to reality. If plans are not revised and reevaluated on an ongoing basis, the plans soon develop a greater divergency with reality and this divergence increases with the passage of time. Without such revision, many nurse decision makers perceive that plans never really apply to the decisions that they make in their daily performance of duties. Organizations have plans at multiple-levels within the organization. At the top of the hierarchy, the plans tend to reflect broader concepts and generally pertain to a longer period of time than plans that are developed lower in the organizational structure. Lower in the structure the objectives tend to be more definite. An interrelatedness and complimentary nature of these plans must exist in order to provide a sense of organizational direction and accomplishment.

STRATEGIC AND TACTICAL PLANNING

In the development of organizational plans, it is necessary to establish the difference between strategic and tactical planning. Some confusion exists among decision makers regarding this matter. In some cases a decision is viewed by one person as strategic, whereas, another individual views the decision as tactical. For purposes of this discussion, strategic planning will refer to longer range planning, and tactical planning will be associated with shorter range planning. Hence, strategic planning is directed toward decisions that will have a longer range and more enduring effect than tactical planning in which the effect is short range and can be modified more easily. For example, the decision by the nurse-manager to recommend the commitment of administration to a highly sophisticated piece of equipment, such as a computerized axial tomography unit, is more difficult to change than the placement of a water cooler for a unit in a certain period of time.

Drucker (1973, p. 125) has defined strategic planning as "the continuous process of making present entrepreneurial (risk-taking) decisions systematically and with the greatest knowledge of their futurity; organizing systematically the efforts needed to carry out these decisions; and measuring the results of these decisions against the expectations through organized systemic feedback."

As this definition states, there are many components in the planning process. It is now necessary to examine the parts of this process.

COMPONENTS OF PLANS

The planning process consists of many components that cannot be considered as a mutually exclusive set, but, rather, they interact and interrelate. For purposes of this discussion and to develop a theoretical framework for future use, the components will be considered as separate parts. Some of these components were discussed in the previous chapter, but the entire component set will be presented to show the total planning process.

Ackoff (1970, p. 6) has defined the five parts of a plan as follows:

1 *Ends:* specification of objectives and goals [Objectives and goals were covered in Chapter 3.]

2 *Means:* selection of policies, programs, procedures and practices by which objectives and goals are to be pursued [These were also covered in Chapter 3.]

3 *Resources:* determination of the types and amounts of resources required, how they are to be generated or acquired and how they are to be allocated to activities [These are covered in Part Three, Section A, Formal Organizing.]

4 *Implementation:* design of decision-making procedures and a way of organizing them so that the plan can be carried out [This area will be covered in Part Four, Section A, Formal Directing.]

5 *Control:* design of a procedure for anticipating or detecting errors in, or failures of, the plan and for preventing or correcting them on a continuing basis [Control will be covered in Part Five, Section A, Formal Controlling.]

All plans do not contain the full set of components that have been listed. However, the above set of components is the minimum for a complete plan.

To illustrate the concept of the development of multilevel plans within the organization and to demonstrate the evolutionary nature of plans over time, the remainder of this discussion will be premised on the basis of a new organization. This approach will help establish a theoretical framework from which ongoing organizations can be evaluated and perhaps better understood.

MULTILEVEL PLANS

The founding board of trustees of a hospital has an overriding and principal purpose. Initially this mission may be merely stated as "wanting to do something in health care in the members' community." As this statement is further refined, the board defines a series of long-range goals. These goals are represented by a series of statements of accomplishments that they wish to achieve over the next few years. These initial statements generally provide the overall direction for the development of the organization through its soon-to-be-developed resources to deliver health care to the community.

The long-range goals collectively constitute the long-range plan of the organization. The plan receives input from numerous individuals and organizations of the community with regard to specific perceived needs for health care delivery. The board, realizing that not all the needs can be met immediately, will prepare plans for each of perhaps the first five years. These plans will be couched in terms of specific objectives to be accomplished within each annual plan. The annual plan interfaces with the long-range plan and should support the general goals as stated.

This process is depicted in Figure 4-1. Based upon available information at the time that these plans are developed, it should be realized that the detailing of the first-year-plan will be significantly greater than the second-year plan and so forth. Throughout the first year, a continuous evaluation of accomplishments will be made, and information will be collected to prepare for the reassessment and reevaluation of the second-year plan for relevancy and the ability of the organization to accomplish the proposed objectives. Thus, a process of reiteration occurs for the second-year plan. This process is shown in Figure 4-2. It will encompass a comparative function between the first-year plan and first-year results for accomplishments and nonaccomplishments including reasons for same. A test of compatibility and possible need for change will occur between the long-range plan and the first-year plan and first-year results. The results of this tripartite analysis will provide input into the proposed

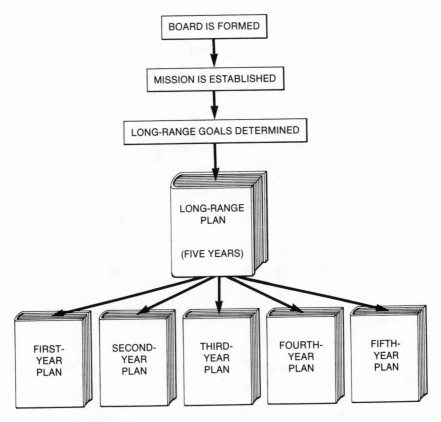

Figure 4-1 Planning Process—Founding Board of Directors

second-year plan including the first-year experience, additional information, and the original second-year plan. This process will continue each year for each proposed annual plan.

As the annual plan is developed, it derives its content from its relationship to the overall direction as indicated in the long-range plan. This process becomes more complex as each department establishes its plan for the year in conjunction with the organizational annual plan. Departments' needs for carrying out their perceived roles are considered. The departmental plans then interface with the overall organizational plan for the proposed year. This concept is depicted in Figure 4-3.

Each of the proposed departmental plans and specific requests therein are then put on a scale of priorities based on scope of projected patient needs, available funding, and other factors. This process results in what the department will have to work with in the upcoming year in terms of personnel and equipment. (This aspect of management will be covered

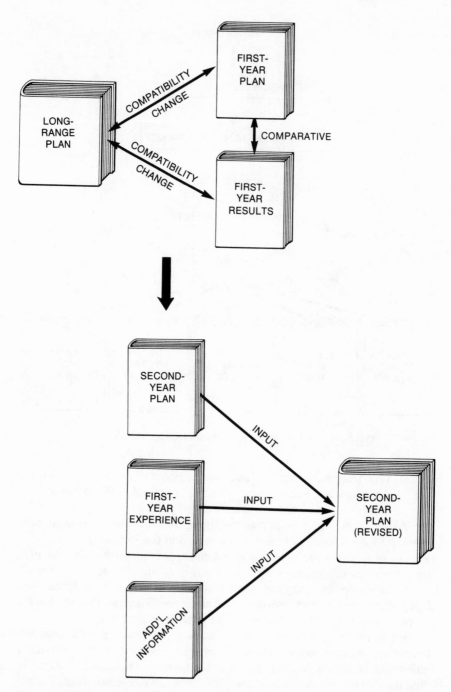

Figure 4-2 Reiteration Process for Subsequent-Year Plans

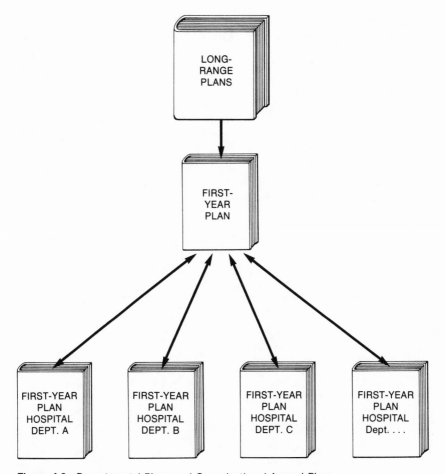

Figure 4-3 Departmental Plans and Organizational Annual Plans

in greater detail under Organizing.) The final decision of priorities is made by the board of directors.

For purposes of our discussion, we will focus on the nursing department. (In some hospital settings, the nursing department is an integral part of what is defined as patient-care systems, which also includes nursing education, social services, and the different specific patient-care areas.)

The nursing department has a series of patient-care areas reporting to it for which it has direct nursing responsibility. These areas include medical, surgical, obstetrics, pediatrics, emergency, critical care, and orthopedics. Within the overall annual plan for the nursing department, the specific patient-care area will develop annual plans for consideration in the overall plan of the nursing department. Note that a protocol and procedures manual should be developed in conjunction with the unit plan and should be revised at least annually. This is illustrated in Figure 4-4.

NURSING CARE PLANS

Once the patient-care unit plans have been approved as they relate to the responsibility of nursing, then the unit supervisor and staff are prepared to begin nursing-care plans.

When the patient has been admitted and a physician's diagnosis made, a nursing assessment or diagnosis is developed, which collectively provides the assessment of the patient's total care needs. At this point a

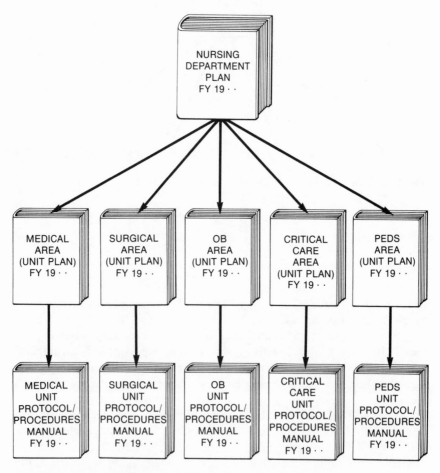

Figure 4-4 Nursing Department Plan and Patient-Care Area Plans

nursing-care plan is developed for each patient including nursing-care objectives, nursing-care means, nursing-care resources, nursing-care implementation (or intervention), and nursing-care control (or review). The process is depicted in Figure 4-5.

The physician diagnosis is concerned with the development of a therapeutic plan that is sometimes referred to as a design for cure. In contrast, the "nursing diagnosis leads to a *plan for nursing care* which is primarily concerned with sustaining, preserving, and conserving the individual's adaptive, defense, and enforcing mechanisms, and with removing or reducing stress or stimuli. The nursing-care plan also includes measures related to the plan for cure (the application and executive of the legal orders of the physician), but its uniqueness resides in its focus upon

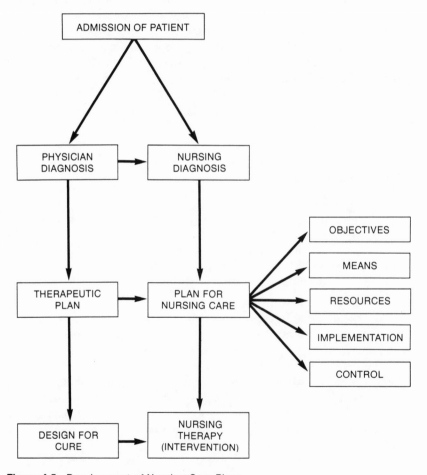

Figure 4-5 Development of Nursing-Care Plans

nursing therapy, those measures directed toward the alleviation of the patient's disease and the modification of his perception of his illness'' (Eckelberry, 1971, p. 50).

A nursing-care plan (NCP) provides a basis or design by which actions can be taken by nurses that are organized into a sequence and progression. The NCP will be written and accessible to those individuals who will care for the patient and family. In most cases the deliverance of the care under the plan is accomplished by many nurses and is a shared activity. As with other plans in the organization, the NCP should be couched with sufficient flexibility to permit change. It must be remembered that the NCP should be dynamic in nature and at the same time be the product of continuing reassessment and objective setting, as well as provide the basis of decisions for action. The benefits of the NCP as it relates to the organizing of resources and their implementation will be covered later.

The NCP then ''is an abstract of data concerning a specific patient— data which is organized in a concise and systematic manner, which facilitates overall medical and nursing goals, and which clearly communicates the nature of the patient's problems and the nature of the related medical and nursing orders'' (Mayers, 1972, p. 13).

The essential components of the NCP according to Mayers (1972, pp. 14–15) are as follows:

Physician's expectations of course of treatment
Nursing criteria for discharge or maintenance
Physician's orders
Usual problems
Unusual problems
Expected outcomes
Prescribed nursing actions
Patient response
Standard care routine

It is essential that nurse-managers be thoroughly familiar with these essential components of the NCP. The understanding of these concepts and the ability to implement them effectively on the unit is necessary to assure the deliverance of quality nursing.

The approach provided by Mayers uses the scientific method in developing the NCP. It is recommended as one of the best resources to obtain an indepth working knowledge of the NCP concept. For the purpose of this discussion, an overview of the components of the NCP will be provided to assist you in the later detailed study of this concept.

Physicians' expectations with regard to the course of treatment is necessary because many times the medical diagnosis does not provide sufficient specificity of expectations. The same diagnosis for two specific patients may not have the same expectations for recovery. Thus, the physician's expectations assist the nurse by providing a reference point for the nursing assessment and can, in many cases, effectively aid the nurse in establishing priorities in nursing care.

The nursing criteria as expressed in terms of outcome criteria allows the nurse to establish measurable patient-centered objectives. A specific target date for attainment must be incorporated as an integral part of the objective of any plan. Objectives are necessary for planning resource use and to ensure the timely deliverance of care. In addition, the objectives provide a mechanism for the evaluation of the nursing care provided. The expected outcome then implies an intended basis for correction of a problem within a specific time.

The listing of patient problems is the first step in securing what barriers must be overcome through care to affect a discharge of the patient. It is important that the problems be segregated into two lists—one for usual problems and one for unusual problems. In the case of usual problems, the unit should develop a manual for protocol and procedures, which is sometimes referred to as standard-care routines. The standard-care routines provide a standard set of nursing activities that are appropriate for the care of patients who are performing and progressing within the limits of expected norms for a specified condition. Once these care routines have been established, the operations of the unit are greatly enhanced. When more standardized nursing care is provided, much time and effort are saved by merely referring to the standardized-care routine in the nursing-care plan. This approach permits the nurse-manager and staff to focus upon the unusual problems that would require considerably more attention to patient needs.

From the identified problems (usual and unusual) prescribed nursing actions (or interventions) can be delineated. These nursing orders would address what, when, and how the nursing care should be delivered.

During the course of the nursing intervention, statements of the patient's responses are obtained. These responses, not technically a part of the NCP, are usually recorded in the nurses' notes and are later used for measurement of progress as perceived by the patient.

Nursing care plans are being used throughout the country. In some cases they have been viewed as merely an exercise. Those nurses who have implemented effective plans are well aware of their advantages. As more and more public concern is expressed over quality of care, the NCP will no longer be viewed as an exercise but rather as a necessity to the deliverance of quality nursing care.

SUMMARY

Formal plans are needed to anticipate future desired results and to prepare for them in advance. The plan as written provides an interim report in the total planning process. The process of planning is ongoing and requires continual reevaluation and reassessment. Thus, a plan must be dynamic by its very nature, and allow for flexibility. This approach to planning ensures the plans' relevancy.

Planning was defined as the specification in advance of goals and means. Means include the planning for resources, implementation strategies, and control mechanisms. It was noted that strategic planning is directed toward decisions that will have a longer range and enduring effect, whereas tactical planning is more concerned with the shorter range and can be modified more easily.

The five components of a plan are ends, means, resources, implementation, and control. The concept of multilevel plans was developed. We noted that the board of directors provides the overall long-range direction for the organization through the long-range plan. This plan provides a series of statements of goals that the organization hopes to accomplish. These goals are broad but realistic, nonquantitative, and have no specified time frame. A series of annual plans is developed from the long-range plan, with specific objectives and time deadlines for accomplishment. These annual plans in general support the goals as delineated in the long-range plan.

Within the framework of the annual plan, a series of departmental plans evolves in concert with the annual organizational plan. A nursing department annual plan was discussed and an explanation given of the various unit plans that are produced for specific care areas. It was noted that each unit provides a written protocol and procedures manual in conjunction with its annual plan.

Each multilevel plan should be reiterated and compared with results for that year. This experiential information, plus additional information, should be used in the revision of the next annual plan.

Consideration was given to nursing care plans (NCPs). We noted that the diagnosis performed by the physician is for the purpose of developing a therapeutic plan as a design for cure, whereas the nursing diagnosis leads to a plan for nursing care that is primarily designed to sustain, preserve, and conserve the patient's adaptive, defensive and enforcing mechanisms and to remove or reduce stress. The NCP provides the basis by which actions can be taken by nurses. We concluded that all plans, including NCP, are dynamic and must be continuously reassessed.

BIBLIOGRAPHY

Ackoff, Russell L. *A Concept of Corporate Planning*. New York: Wiley-Interscience, 1970.
Chambers, W. "Nursing Diagnosis." *American Journal of Nursing*. 62 (1962): 102–104.

Drucker, Peter F. *The Practice of Management*. New York: Harper & Row, 1954.

_____. *Management: Tasks, Responsibilities and Practices*. New York: Harper & Row, 1973.

Eckelberry, Grace K. *Administration of Comprehensive Nursing Care*. New York: Appleton-Century-Crofts, 1971.

Flippo, Edwin B. *Management: A Behavioral Approach;* 2nd ed. Boston: Allyn & Bacon, 1970.

Korn, Thora. *Nursing Team Leadership,* 2nd ed. Philadelphia: Saunders, 1966.

Little, D., and Carnevali, D. *Nursing Care Planning*. Philadelphia: Lippincott, 1969.

Mayers, Marlene Glover. *A Systematic Approach to the Nursing Care Plan*. New York: Appleton-Century-Crofts, 1972.

Phaneuf, Maria C. *The Nursing Audit: Profile for Excellence*. New York: Appleton-Century-Crofts, 1972.

Perlin, Martin S. "Current Practices in Long-Range Planning." *Hospitals,* vol. 46, no. 17 (September 1, 1972): 62–65.

Sayles, Leonard R., and Chandler, Margaret K. *Managing Large Systems: Organizations for the Future*. New York: Harper & Row, 1971.

Schleh, Edward C. *Management by Results: The Dynamics of Profitable Management*. New York: McGraw-Hill, 1961.

Webber, James B., and Dula, Martha A. "Effective Planning Committees for Hospitals." *Harvard Business Review,* vol. 52, no. 3 (May-June 1974): 133–142.

Wiley, Loy. "Juggling Patients on the Head of a Pin or How Much Can a Mere Mortal Do?" *Nursing '75* (December 1975): 55–57.

Behavioral Influences on Planning

Chapter 5

The Individual Nurse

By the very nature of his or her education, the individual nurse is concerned for the patient. Much emphasis is placed on the patient's needs and problems, as it should be. Nurses work hard to understand these problems and implement mechanisms to assist the patient to reduce or eliminate them.

Research by many psychologists and sociologists has shown that our understanding of others is only as great as the understanding we have of our own needs as human beings. Thus, the ability to manage other human beings will rest upon our ability to understand ourselves. From our foundation will evolve our basic understanding of human beings and how we will approach them and work with them in carrying out our managerial responsibility.

EMPHASIS ON THE INDIVIDUAL IN NURSING

The movement toward greater emphasis on the individual in nursing has occurred over the past half century. Wilson (1959–1960, p. 177) noted that:

already in the 1920s there were undoubtedly large metropolitan hospitals in which the physician's autonomy was being curtailed by the expanding formal bureaucratic *desiderata,* the proliferation of paramedical specialties, an increasing awareness and demandingness of community and patient. . . . [the physician's] role as unchallenged master, what might be conceived as a charismatic role, is changing. No longer do nurses open doors for him or spring to their feet when he enters a room; . . . no longer, even, do his sophisticated patients grant him quite the omniscience they once did.

The leading force for change was the growth of specialization in medical practice. As the autonomy of the individual physician was reduced due to this proliferation of specialties, so the complexity of medical practice within each specialty became a reality with increased use of technological advances. These advances produce a virtual team of nurses, support personnel, and equipment necessary to provide quality patient care. As a result of these developments, the role of the nurse greatly increased with the need for increased knowledge and skills, which the profession of nursing is earnestly working to meet. Throughout this time, nurses' roles have continued to expand as they became a more dominant force in the delivery of care to patients. Today, nurses are charged with the coordination of the total patient-care needs.

Thus, from the time of the almshouses, nurses have gone from a minimal subservient role to the physician to key members of the health team coordinating the needs of the patient. In the early years management did not accurately put in perspective the importance of the nurses' role in the hospital setting. This situation was evidenced by low wages and poor working conditions. The nurses' needs were often ignored, and frustration prevailed. The primary causes for this development were managers' ignorance and the overriding importance of hospital objectives over individual nurse needs.

This inappropriate management of the individual took place over a long period of time, throughout which nurses have been working to correct the situation. Some inroads have been made, but much work remains to be accomplished. The 1930's produced some change in federal law permitting employees to join unions. The National Labor Relations (Wagner) Act of 1935 established the first national labor policy of protecting the rights of workers to organize and to elect their representatives for collective bargaining. This act provided for unionization of hospital workers. However, in 1947 the Taft-Hartley Act amended the Wagner Act to remove hospitals from coverage under this law. In 1974 following years of lobbying, the American Nurses' Association (ANA) was able to secure the passage of legislation that removed nonprofit hospitals from exemption under the Taft-Hartley Act. We can assume that this amendment will lead to increased activity of unions in hospitals.

It must be remembered that these laws evolve from the attitudinal changes in society. Nursing management and hospital administrations must recognize these shifts in society. The private sector must study these human problems and provide solutions before solutions are imposed by society that feels not enough has been done for the individual. It is far better to do some preventive management rather than wait for the situation to reach an acute stage of development.

Thus, nurse-managers must be aware of basic needs of individuals in order to understand sufficiently the behavior of employees on a unit. Managers must understand that employees are people, too; they must not assume that all people are alike. They are not; consequently, they act as individuals. Individual differences do exist. Individuals possess certain needs that they are continually working to satisfy, and the lack of satisfaction is expressed through various levels of maladjustment. Many individuals demonstrate frustration when they cannot find means of satisfying their needs. Frustration can be expressed in various ways—through aggression, regression, fixation, or even resignation. In order to better understand relative levels of maladjustment, it is essential that nurse-managers be aware of individuals' need patterns.

HIERARCHY OF NEEDS

Psychologists have identified many human needs. Most believe that the basic physiological needs are the first ones that must be satisfied. Abraham Maslow (1954) developed a hierarchy of needs that has received wide acceptance among managers throughout this country. Essentially, Maslow established five levels of needs that an individual must satisfy:

1. Physiologic needs
2. Security or safety needs
3. Social needs
4. Ego needs
5. Self-fulfillment needs

The hierarchy-of-needs theory indicates that the individual must satisfy the lower level needs (such as physiologic and security) before higher level needs (ego and self-fulfillment) can be satisfied. Once a need level has been reasonably satisfied, then the individual is motivated to satisfy a higher level need. This process is unending and continues from birth to death.

At the lowest level of an individual's needs, but of paramount importance when they are not met, are physiologic needs. Thus, an individual must have water, food, air, and shelter from the elements. When these basic needs are not being met—that is, when the individual is hungry the individual's needs for love, status, recognition are unimportant. But when an individual eats regularly, he or she is motivated to meet a higher level need. An essentially satisfied need cannot be a motivation of behavior. Thus, when basic physiologic needs are reasonably met, needs at the next higher level—namely, security or safety needs—then dominate and act to motivate the individual toward accomplishing the higher level need.

This second level of needs reflects the desires of the individual to assure that the satisfaction of needs on the first level will continue over time. These needs are for protection against danger and threat. Included in this category is fear of deprivation. Hence, the individual as an employee is performing in a somewhat dependent state and as such is subject to management decisions that may arouse a considerable degree of uncertainty about position and, in some cases, continued employment.

Once the individual has met the basic physiologic needs and feels reasonably secure that these needs will continue to be satisfied, then he or she is motivated to meet the needs of the third level. The third level of needs is social in nature. One has needs for giving and receiving love, for acceptance and association, and for belonging to someone. Nurse-managers are aware of the existence of these needs but many times erroneously view these needs as representing a barrier to the efficient and smooth operation of a unit. Numerous studies have shown that a cohesive group of workers may, under proper conditions, produce a more effective working situation than where such cohesion does not exist. In some nursing units nurse-managers with an overriding fear of group hostility will attempt to direct individuals in a way that precludes the development of cohesive groups. In this way, managers may deprive individuals of the satisfaction of social needs. Too often, this type of nurse-manager behavior will elicit individual responses of anger, antagonism, resistance, and general lack of cooperation. Hence, it is necessary that managers provide an environment that does not prevent the satisfaction of these needs.

The fourth level of needs is ego needs. These needs refer to an individual's self-esteem—namely, achievement, competence, knowledge, and self-confidence. In addition, the ego needs relate to respect from others, appreciation, recognition, and status. The impact of nurse-managers is not as great at this level as at social-needs level. The individual must be so motivated that competence and knowledge can be secured and achievement demonstrated. Managers can quite appropriately encourage individuals to pursue these attainments, and if individuals do, in fact, accomplish them, then managers can demonstrate appreciation and recognition and can assist in the attainment of status for the individual. These needs do not usually become prevalent until the physiologic, security, and social needs have generally been satisfied.

The fifth and final level of need is self-fulfillment. This level addresses the realizing of one's potential, the need for being creative, and the need for continued self-improvement and development. Usually, the great amount of time and energy expended by the individual in meeting the lower level needs leaves little time to devote to the satisfaction of self-fulfillment needs.

An overview of this hierarchy of needs would seem to indicate that in a pragmatic sense the individual is probably never fully satisfied at any level of need. However, if the individual perceives that a need level is reasonably satisfied, then it cannot be considered as a basis for motivation. Thus, the needs that have not been met are the primary motivators of behavior.

CONCEPT OF SELF

In addition to needs, an individual has certain values and abilities. The composition and importance of these needs, values, and abilities provide the individual's self-concept. Carl Rogers (1959) describes self as relating to the centrality or peripheral nature of the individual's needs, values, and abilities. In drawing on the work of Rogers, Argyris (1964, p. 23) stated that:

> the sociocultural matrix in which the individual is embedded has an important influence on the development of these factors. Through the parents, the child begins to learn about the norms of the culture. The specific needs, values, and abilities that he develops will be highly influenced by these cultural norms. . . . The unique integration of these needs or values and abilities into an organized pattern that is functionally meaningful for the individual represents the individual's personality or self.

It is important that managers be aware of this concept. Essentially, it is composed of two aspects: one the individual is aware of, namely the self-concept, and the other refers to the unconscious portions of self. It seems reasonable to assume that the more one is aware of self, the greater the probability for understanding of self and influence and control of behavior. Thus, effective nurse-managers should provide mechanisms in the working environment that will assist individuals in the understanding of themselves.

PERSONALITY AND MATURATION

Argyris (1957) has developed some concepts relating an individual's personality to maturity. As mentioned earlier, an individual's personality is nurtured from childhood to adulthood by the sociocultural matrix that exists throughout life. The maturation process, itself, produces changes in the individual as he or she becomes older. The following observations by Argyris are based on the premise that as one becomes chronologically older, he or she generally tends to move along each continuum from infancy to adulthood, and he developed these observations with regard to aspects of maturity of the individual over time:

1 Development from a state of passivity as an infant to a state of increasing activity as an adult
2 Development from a state of dependence on others as an infant to a state of relative independence as an adult
3 Development from a state of being capable of behaving only in a few ways as an infant to being capable of behaving in many different ways as an adult
4 Development from having erratic, casual, shallow, and quickly dropped interests as an infant to having deeper interests as an adult
5 Development from having a short time perspective as an infant to having a much longer time perspective as an adult
6 Development from being in a subordinate position as an infant to aspiring to occupy an equal and/or superordinate position as an adult
7 Development from a lack of awareness of self as an infant to awareness and control over self as an adult (p. 50)

These aspects are of extreme interest to managers in viewing the placement of various individuals on each continuum. Such identifications are meaningful in understanding some types of behavior and offer a challenge to managers who wish to provide a working environment conducive to helping individuals in the maturation process. The environmental setting and attitude that you as a manager bring to the unit will reflect your own predispositions with regard to the basic nature of individuals.

BASIC NATURE OF INDIVIDUALS

McGregor (1960) studied and observed managers in many settings and environments throughout his lifetime. The key question that McGregor raised in his book *The Human Side of Enterprise* was, "What are your assumptions (implicit as well as explicit) about the most effective way to manage people?" (p. 511) He demonstrated his points through the use of the following example, which depicts management as moving ahead without examination of assumption, and how this practice can lead to management behavior that is inconsistent:

A manager, for example, states that he delegates his subordinates. When asked, he expresses assumptions such as, "People need to learn to take responsibility" or "Those closer to the situation can make the best decisions." However, he has arranged to obtain a constant flow of detailed information about the behavior of his subordinates, and he uses this information to police their behavior and to "second guess" their decisions. He says, "I am held responsible, so I need to know what is going on." He sees no inconsistency in his behavior, nor does he recognize some other assumptions which are implicit: "People can't be trusted," or "They can't really make as good decisions as I can."

With one hand, and in accord with certain assumptions, he delegates; with the other, and in line with other assumptions, he takes actions which have the effect of nullifying his delegation. Not only does he fail to recognize the inconsistencies involved, but if faced with them he is likely to deny them. (p. 7)

It is interesting to note that in the continua that have been described by Argyris, managers tend to establish environments and attitudes that support more of the infancy side of the continuum than the adult side. With this type of setting, it would not be surprising to see an individual express more childlike behavior than might have been expected.

As a result of McGregor's experiences of working with and observing managerial behavior, he developed two theories about the assumptions about human motivation (McGregor, 1960, pp. 34–35, 47–48):

  1 *Theory X* which assumes that people dislike work and must be coerced, controlled, and heavily directed toward the goals of the organization. The individual does not want to assume responsibility.
  2 *Theory Y* which assumes that people have an intrinsic interest in their work, are self-motivated, are self-directed, and seek responsibility.

McGregor's concept of Theory Y as espousing a more participative form of management provided a considerable impact on insights to improving the effectiveness of organizations. Following the dissemination of McGregor's work, many organizations developed management-development programs to train managers in the concepts of more participative management.

More recently, Morse and Lorsch (1975) wrote that many managers believed Theory Y to be the only feasible approach to management as a result of McGregor's work. In "Beyond Theory Y," Morse and Lorsch propose that a contingency or situational approach is perhaps most relevant to developing a productive organization. They imply that the most critical dimension is to establish the best fit of organizational tasks and individuals. They indicate from their research that the appropriate fit appears to develop a "competence motivation," which occurs regardless of organizational style used by management.

Morse's and Lorsch's approach of looking at how the individual and the organization interface, interact, and conflict will provide the basis of the next chapter.

SUMMARY

The individual nurse is concerned for the patient's needs and problems. The understanding we have about others is only as great as the extent of the understanding that we have of our own needs as human beings. From our own foundation will evolve our basic nature as human beings and how we will carry out our own managerial responsibility.

We noted that over the past 50 years there has been a greater emphasis on the individual in nursing that had not been true prior to this period. Nurses worked in almshouses in a minimal subservient role to physicians. This role has changed substantially for many reasons: the proliferation of medical specialties resulting from a team approach to health care delivery; the work of the ANA to remove exemptions for nonprofit hospitals under the Taft-Hartley Act, and the attitudinal changes about the importance of the individual as a person that have occurred and are occurring in society.

We also noted that it is necessary to realize that employees are people, too. We cannot assume that all people are alike. They are individuals. Hence, it is imperative to realize that individual differences exist, that individuals have certain needs, and that they are continually working to satisfy those needs.

We reviewed the work of Maslow in which he developed a configuration of needs for all individuals. The configuration consists of five levels ranging from basic physiologic needs to self-fulfillment needs. An overview of this concept makes it appear that an individual is probably never fully satisfied at any level of need. However, when a need level is reasonably satisfied, it cannot be considered as a basis for motivation.

The concept of self as espoused by Carl Rogers was related to needs and was integrated through the work of Argyris, which discussed the unique integration of needs or values and abilities into a configuration that represents the individual's personality.

We reviewed the work of Argyris regarding the concepts of relating an individual's personality to maturity. A framework evolved that permits managers to place various individuals conceptually on the continuums of maturity to assist in the understanding of behavior. We noted that the environmental setting and attitude that managers bring to the unit will reflect their own predispositions with regard to the basic nature of individuals and will most likely affect the behavior of others.

We discussed McGregor's concepts of Theory X and Theory Y, and we noted that Theory X assumes that people dislike work, must be coerced and controlled with much direction, whereas Theory Y assumes that people have an intrinsic interest in their work and that they are self-motivated and self-directed while seeking responsibility.

Finally, we examined the recent work of Morse and Lorsch. In "Beyond Theory Y" they propose that the theory is not the sole answer to a management approach to individuals. Instead, they propose a contingency or situation concept, which addresses the need to fit organizational tasks with individuals properly. This concept tends to develop a "competence motivation" that enhances organizational effectiveness regardless of the organization style used.

BIBLIOGRAPHY

Argyris, Chris. *Personality and Organization*. New York: Harper & Row, 1957.
———*Integrating the Individual and the Organization*. New York: Wiley, 1964.
Krawleski, John E. "Collective Bargaining Among Professional Employees." *Hospital Administration,* vol. 19, no. 3 (Summer 1974): 30–41.
Maslow, Abraham. *Motivation and Personality*. New York: Harper, 1954.
McGregor, Douglas. *The Human Side of Enterprise*. New York: McGraw-Hill, 1960.
———. *Leadership and Motivation*. Cambridge, Mass.: M.I.T. Press, 1960.
Morse, John J., and Lorsch, Jay W. "Beyond Theory Y." *Harvard Business Review on Management*. New York: Harper & Row, 1975.
Panosh, Michael. "Unionization and Collective Bargaining by Registered Nurses." Unpublished Ph.D. dissertation, University of Wisconsin, Madison, 1973.
Pointer, Dennis D. "How the 1974 Taft-Hartley Amendments Will Affect Health Care Facilities." *Hospital Progress* (October 1974): 68–70.
Rogers, Carl. "A Theory of Therapy, Personality, and Interpersonal Relations as Developed in the Client-Centered Framework." In Sigmund Koch (Ed.) *Psychology: A Study for Science,* vol. 3, edited by Sigmund Koch. New York: McGraw-Hill, 1959.
Wilson, Robert N. "The Physician's Changing Hospital Role." *Human Organization,* vol. 18, no. 4 (Winter 1959–1960): 177–183.

Chapter 6

The Individual Nurse and Organizations

Maslow aptly noted that individuals have needs that must be satisfied. When people approach a new employment situation, there are many unknowns. The nurse faces many factors that in his or her own mind are not settled. For purposes of this discussion, we will consider a new employment situation. This type of situation probably best exemplifies the interactions between the individual and the organization. The greatest amount of adaptation usually occurs during this period of time.

THE NURSE—A NEW EMPLOYEE

Nurses as individuals join an organization, usually a hospital, and become employees of the institution. When they are first employed, they usually have certain expectations about the institution. In addition, the institution has expectations concerning the new employee who will be working on the nursing unit. For the present, let us look at the situation from the new employee's point of view.

Certainly, the views the employees bring to the situation will vary considerably depending on many factors related to cultural background, education and experience. Individual nurses will look to the organization to provide mechanisms for satisfaction of the following needs:

• *Compensation* The employee will expect to receive pay for hours of work given to the organization. The level of pay should be equivalent with other nurses having similar backgrounds and experience. This pay will permit satisfaction of some basic physiologic and safety needs.

• *Job security* The employee would hope that the new position will be stable and will be in existence for a good period of time. In the past this has not been a great problem for nursing positions. However, layoffs and elimination of some positions have occurred recently on an isolated basis in different parts of the country. These situations resulted primarily from administrations' attempts to affect cost containment. A safe environment is part of the employee's need for security.

• *Association and acceptance* The employee will seek associations with professional colleagues in the new environment. When established, these relationships assist the employee in feeling comfortable in a health setting with other employees of similar education, experience, and motivations for delivering quality patient care. In addition, as the nurse performs well on the unit, the association relationships will expand to include acceptance. In some organizations the development of relationships over a long period of time may act to retard the ready acceptance of a new colleague. This period of time prior to acceptance varies widely.

• *Recognition* As the employee continues to perform well in the nursing unit, acceptance becomes greater as colleagues and others recognize well-done work. This recognition can be expressed in many ways from nonverbal communication to a letter from the director of nursing commending the nurse for an outstanding contribution to patient care in the hospital. Recognition of any kind is a positive factor for the individual's ego. With competent leadership that deals fairly with employees, the credibility of such recognition is greatly enhanced. This competency factor coupled with built-in opportunities for advancement will provide an additional motivational basis for high achievement.

Thus, it becomes quite evident that the new nurse employee enters the employment situation with a myriad of hopes and expectations of the organization. However, the new employee is not the only one with such expectations. Employees with many years with the organization have certain hopes and expectations. The probability of those expectations becoming reality are generally better known by the employee with more experience with that particular organization. In all cases the new employee is interacting with other employees and the organization. The extent to which these interactions are more favorable than unfavorable will determine, to a great degree, the length of time of employment. If more employees interact unfavorably than favorably, there is usually a measurable increase in employee turnover.

NURSE/ORGANIZATIONAL INTERFACE

Through its planning process, the organization developed a series of organization goals and objectives. In addition, nurses have personal goals and aspirations that they bring to the organizational setting. The relative congruence and compatibility of organizational needs and individual nurse needs will determine to a great extent the "goodness of fit." The greater the congruency, the better the fit; likewise, the lesser the congruency, the worse the fit.

Problems of good fit can come from many sources. Perhaps the most obvious source of problems comes from a direct conflict of organizational objectives and individual needs. From the nurse's standpoint, the situation can occur when a concerted effort is being made to deliver quality nursing care to patients in a unit of high-census and high-acuity patients, and administration states that there can be no new additions to the staff. In this case, nurses feel frustrated about not being able to do the kind of job they feel is necessary to deliver quality nursing care. The administration, on the other hand, is probably trying to work within the limits of a tight budget approved by the board of trustees or some rate-setting commission. Thus, a direct conflict can occur in which the nurses feel that nursing care is being hindered by administrative decisions. If the situation continues for a considerable period of time, nurses will come into direct conflict with the administration and, if they get no support, may seek another environment. Sometimes these conditions of conflict exist because there is a lack of understanding of goals. Many times the manner in which the problem is approached by one or both parties increases the level of conflict. On the other hand, some practice of diplomacy appropriately delivered can secure needed results.

Another source of "goodness-of-fit" problems is the manner in which management approaches its planning process. If management uses a traditional planning process, it can reasonably expect nurse resistance when it is time to implement the plan. The traditional planning process is totally developed at the top of the organization without input from nurses. The nurses are then expected to work under the *imposed* conditions. For many years, nurses were told to accept and work within the imposed conditions. As time has progressed and society changed to greater openness, the extent of outright acceptance of imposed conditions has diminished.

The effect of this change has been positive. As a result of the nurses' resistance to the imposed (changed) conditions, supervisors and administrators began seeking ways to secure greater acceptance and less resistance to change. Many times supervisors described this as being more cooperative. From the individual nurse's standpoint, the resistance was not solely to fight change but rather to attempt to increase the effectiveness of the working environment so that the best nursing care could be delivered to the patients. At the same time, few managers are naïve enough to believe that every plan developed would be implemented without some modification. However, managers must remember that the individual nurses on the unit have personalities and that collectively human personalities show great diversity. Consequently, behavior cannot be programmed.

Many managers have found that using a more participative approach to planning can increase acceptance because of increased involvement. This approach does not guarantee that some resistance will not occur, but it does help in the overall implementation. In addition to the problem of overcoming resistance to change through a more participative approach, plans developed by people who will implement them can produce better plans. The resulting plans can be more detailed, and in many cases, some vague areas are clarified and unforeseen problems are identified.

The more traditional planning processes can produce plans that tend to limit participation, greatly structure roles and functions, provide little room for individual initiative, and result many times in employee apathy. The individual does not identify with, or relate to, the resulting plans due to the lack of participation. In addition, the extent of structuring of roles and positions acts to stifle individual freedom and initiative while producing a threat to the individual's ego. The lack of involvement usually reduces understanding and the rationales that were the basis for the development of the plans. As plans are further delineated, policies and procedures evolve that affect nurses even more directly. Without an understanding of the plans, these individuals will not understand the policies and procedures. This situation is further exacerbated because of the problem nurses have in attempting to see how policies and procedures interrelate and support objectives as specified in the plans. In the end, the traditional approach tends greatly to reduce the nurses' ability to secure gratification of their individual needs as promulgated by Maslow. The physiologic and safety needs can usually be met under this approach, but there is little hope of satisfying the higher level needs such as association, acceptance, recognition, and achievement.

ORGANIZATIONAL ADAPTATION AND EMPLOYEE MOTIVATION

As we have seen, the working environment and management approach to developing and sustaining that environment is important for cooperation, for reducing resistance to change, and for providing mechanisms for satisfaction of individual needs. It is becoming more and more apparent to managers that compensation and benefit programs alone will not provide a quality environment without consideration of the human factors at work in that environment.

Walton (1975, p. 359) states that "regardless of how we approach the issue of the quality of work life, we must acknowledge the diversity of human preference—diversity relating to culture, social class, family rearing, education, and personality." It is quite clear that management must develop appropriate mechanisms that will permit flexibility whereby individual differences can be fused into the work environment. The accommodation of such differences should assist in the assimilation of the individual into the organizational setting. To the extent that this accommodation can be achieved, the more likely that the "goodness of fit" of the individual and the organization within reasonable bounds can become a reality.

The majority of the discussion thus far has addressed the Maslow's need structure of the individual and the goals of the organization. But do we know what motivates employees?

Frederick Herzberg (1968) has studied this area. Initially, Herzberg establishes the hypothesis that "the psychology of motivation is tremendously complex, and what has been unraveled with any degree of assurance is small indeed" (p. 53). This modest statement is somewhat misleading because the theory draws from the original research and has been replicated in many settings. "At least 16 other investigations, using a wide variety of populations (including some in communist countries), have since been completed, making the original research one of the most replicated sudies in the field of job attitudes" (Herzberg, 1968, p. 56). The original underlying premise addresses a single continuum ranging from satisfaction to dissatisfaction. However, the research findings showed that "factors involved in producing job satisfaction (and motivation) are separate and distinct from factors that lead to job dissatisfaction" (Herzberg, 1968, p. 56).

Herzberg proposes that two continuums of separate factors exist. One group of factors was called "hygienic" constituted a continuum with end points of dissatisfaction to no satisfaction and included such factors as company policy, supervision, relationship with supervisor, salary, and security. The second continuum of factors was called "motivators." These factors ranged from no job satisfaction to job satisfaction. "Motivators" included achievement, recognition, work itself, responsibility, and achievement. It is of interest to note that the "hygienic" factors are basically extrinsic to the job (environment), whereas the "motivators" are intrinsic and related to the content of the job itself. Thus, "motivators" provide the principal cause for job satisfaction, whereas "hygienic" factors were the principal cause of dissatisfaction. Some of the groups of employees included in these investigations were professional women, military officers, engineers, housekeepers, accountants, professional nurses, and others.

Drawing on the results of this research, the nurse managers would conclude that an increase in compensation, fringe benefits, and a more understanding supervisor will not motivate staff but will instead reduce these possible areas of staff dissatisfaction. Herzberg (1975) has suggested that a process of "job enrichment" should be considered. Basically, job enrichment attempts to enrich the work through effective use of personnel. This approach is in opposition to traditional management theory, which attempted to rationalize the work in order to increase efficiency. At this stage, from a very pragmatic point of view, is it reasonable to assume that all positions can be redesigned to incorporate such aspects of enrichment? Certainly, many positions that have been rigid for some time might benefit greatly from some facelifting. However, from a total organizational standpoint, it may not be feasible.

INDIVIDUAL DIFFERENCES, INDIVIDUAL ADAPTATIONS, AND EXTERNAL JOB FACTORS

Thus far, the discussion has centered on the needs of the individual and how the organization might adapt itself to the individual. Certainly, individual differences should be recognized, and the organization should make a concerted effort to incorporate flexibility whenever possible. However, some writers have produced additional thoughts and insights regarding many assumptions that have been previously stated.

Is it reasonable to assume that all employees wish to mature in the sense described by Argyris? Will all employees feel a sense of creativity and be self-motivated and self-controlled as proposed in Theory Y? Will job enrichment truly motivate employees, or will it be viewed as an additional work burden if more responsibilities are added to an existing job?

Dubin (1961, pp. 60–61) has suggested that individual employees can and will adjust to varying work environments. He contends that employees will adapt to structured job situations identified with the traditional management approach. Dubin feels that most employees are basically indifferent toward work and, further, that they will probably seek fulfillment outside the work setting.

In a later work, Strauss (1963, p. 70) raised questions regarding the generalizations of employees. He believes that the need structures do not necessarily apply to rank-and-file workers but more likely apply to highly educated professional employees. These findings were later supported by research that indicated a positive correlation between job structure and need satisfaction, particularly for higher level needs in the Maslow hierarchy (Sexton, 1968, pp. 3–7).

Morse and Lorsch (1975) propose that a contingency or situational approach is perhaps the most relevant alternate to Theory Y, whereby the most critical dimension is considered—the best fit of organizational tasks and individuals. This best fit appears to develop a "competence motivation" for the employee and is most relevant to developing a productive organization.

Douglas Sherwin (1975, p. 685) recently addressed the following question:

> "What will happen if we do not find a way to let our employees meet their psychological needs on the job?" He notes that "Theory Y remains but a potential . . . Theory X behavior is what we observe all around. . . . Can we really expect much for a Theory-Y style of managing if it is simply overlaid onto assumptions of organizing that prevent the employee from meeting his psychological needs. . . . Environment selects behavior, and the . . . organization selects Theory X behavior . . .

Sherwin proposed a new approach that is based on creating an organization in which the concept of change has been incorporated as an integral part. He states, "We need a new concept of employees; we need to regard them as discrete, versatile resource units, able to make contributions where needed in the organization, rather than as fixed components of particular divisions and hierarchies." Sherwin supports the employee as the change agent. He notes that "when one thinks about it, it is strange that 'resistance to change' is what is reported by observers of organizational behavior when actually 'change' presents the best chance employees have to satisfy their psychological needs! The key to this paradox is that change is great when you are its agent; it is only bad when you are its object" (Sherwin, 1975, p. 684).

Thus, Dubin, Strauss, Morse and Lorsch, and Sherwin provide some very interesting thoughts with regard to the original writings of Argyris, McGregor, Maslow, and Herzberg. These thoughts have questioned some of the generalizations of the maturation concept, Theory Y, the Herzberg theory, and the Maslow theory. The points that have been raised perhaps clarify further and amend some of the original theories. But in any event, all of the approaches have caused the role of the individual to be advanced and considered by the managers of today and tomorrow.

SUMMARY

We examined the interface of the nurse as an employee, and we reviewed the role of the new nurse employee with various expectations. The needs of the individual that might be satisfied by the organization were explored, including compensation, job security, association and acceptance, and recognition. We noted that employees who have been in the institution for some time have many of the same needs as new employees. However, the probability of those expectations becoming reality are generally better known by the employee with more experience with that particular organization.

We examined the sources of problems of goodness of fit. The goodness-of-fit concept relates to the congruency and compatibility of individual goals with organizational goals. The greater the congruency, the better the fit; the lesser the congruency, the worse the fit. The first problem source of direct conflict was noted through a quality of nursing-care/cost-containment situation. We observed that many times the manner in which the problem is approached by one or both parties can increase the level of conflict. An added source of problems results from the way management approaches its planning process. If this process is done in a traditional way, resistance usually occurs because nurses are expected to work under the imposed conditions that evolve from the planning process. The general acceptance of imposed conditions appears to have diminished over time.

Management has sought out ways to reduce resistance to change and increase the acceptability of plans. Greater acceptance appears under conditions of greater employee involvement in the development of those plans.

As a result, management has found that using a more participative approach to planning can increase acceptance of the plans and the process itself. The total elimination of resistance cannot be guaranteed. The resulting plans using this approach can be more detailed, and in many cases, some vague areas can be clarified and some unforeseen problems identified.

We examined the negative aspects of the traditional planning process. These aspects included the limited effect on participation, greatly structured roles and functions, limited room for individual initiative, and possible increased employee apathy. The policies and procedures that evolve from this type of process are implemented without employee understanding. The problem is further exacerbated because nurses do not know the rationale behind the policies and procedures and how they interrelate with objectives as specified in the plans. This planning process provides little hope for the satisfaction of higher level needs of association, acceptance, recognition, and achievement.

Various aspects of organizational adaptation and employee motivation were examined. The concept of accommodating individual differences in the organizational environment as a catalyst in the assimilation of the individual in the environment was considered. We discussed the work of Herzberg on motivation, which resulted in the two-continuum concept of "motivation" and "hygiene" factors, and we considered the concept of job enrichment as a possible factor to assist in employee motivation.

We further suggested that employees can and will adapt to structured situations. Furthermore, the challenge to the generalizations of applicability of need structures was presented through the work of Strauss, and we reviewed the contingency approach to goodness of fit by Morse and Lorsch. Finally, we examined the work of Sherwin, which advocated a new approach to organizations, providing the concept of change as an integral part of the organizational structure. Sherwin sees the employee as the change agent.

BIBLIOGRAPHY

Dubin, Robert. *Human Relations in Administration,* 2nd ed. Englewood Cliffs, N.J.: Prentice-Hall, 1961.

Herzberg, Frederick. "One More Time: How Do You Motivate Employees?" *Harvard Business Review,* vol. 46, no. 1 (January–February 1968): 53–62.

Morse, John J., and Lorsch, Jay W. "Beyond Theory Y." *Harvard Business Review on Management.* New York: Harper & Row, 1975.

Sexton, William. "Industrial Work: Who Calls It Psychologically Devastating?" *Management of Personnel Quarterly,* vol. 6, no. 4 (Winter 1968): 2–8.

Sherwin, Douglas S. "Strategy for Winning Employee Commitment." *Harvard Business Review on Management.* New York: Harper & Row, 1975.

Strauss, George. "The Personality vs. Organization Theory." In *Individualism and Big Business,* edited by Leonard Sayles. New York: McGraw-Hill, 1963.

Walton, Richard E. "Improving the Quality of Work Life." *Harvard Business Review of Management.* New York: Harper & Row, 1975.

Part Three

Organizing in Nursing

Part Three provides concepts of organizing in nursing. We will review the functions of nursing, examine the organizing process, and consider the structure of organizations in nursing (Section A). Then we will review the behavioral influences on the formal organizing process, including informal aspects of organizations, sociopolitical forces in nursing as well as the effects of specialization (Section B).

In Chapter 7, we will consider the organic functions of a hospital and review the functions of nursing care. The concepts of primary and secondary functions will be covered in addition to functions and their relationship to organizational maturation. We will consider the need for functional balance as it relates to functionalizational and managerial span of control.

Chapter 8 provides background and insight into the organizing process in nursing. We will review concepts of design and personnel resources. In addition, tools for the nurse-manager are covered including responsibility, authority, and accountability.

Chapter 9 examines the structure of organizations in nursing including structural delivery systems, structural considerations, and diagnosis of structural problems. The delivery systems examined are the case-method system, functional-method system, team-method system, and the primary-care-method system.

In Chapter 10 we will review the infomal aspects of organizations. Included in the discussion of informal aspects are informal groups, rationale for informal groups, and the management of informal groups.

Chapter 11 provides insight into the sociopolitical forces at work in nursing. Topics covered include status systems, authority and power systems, and organizational political systems.

In the final chapter on organizing, the effects of specialization in nursing are reviewed. We will examine the following concepts: functional differentiation, role of the clinical nurse specialist, nurse-manager and specialization, and the integration of specialists into the milieu of the unit.

Formal Organizing

Chapter 7

Functions in Nursing

A common statement heard on most nursing units: "Today we have got to get organized." Nurse-managers or unit staff members who express this view are venting frustrations about the fact that unit is not perceived as functioning in a smooth and systematic manner. This statement usually applies to the need to satisfy a short-term need within the period of that particular shift. The action proposed is usually needed, and quite frequently it is needed on a daily basis. The question then becomes "Why do we have to get organized every day?" The problem is that perhaps we are treating the symptoms and not the cause.

Many of the problems that occur in a unit come from the way the unit was organized. What we perceive as the need to organize are actually the aberrations of the basic foundation. Therefore, it is imperative that we address the question of basic organization, so that we may understand and perhaps correct the aberrations that we observe on the unit.

In these three chapters we will cover the concept of organizing, including functions in nursing, the organizing process in nursing, and the structure of organizations in nursing.

ORGANIZING

As we have seen in Part Two, goals and objectives are developed by organizations, and they are incorporated into plans. We examined some of the behavioral influences on planning, and we identified some of the needs of individual nurses and how they interfaced with the organization. Now we must see how the organization is developed to provide the necessary mechanisms to carry out the plans.

Flippo (1970, p.4) has defined organizing as "the process of establishing relationships among these components [of personnel, physical factors, and functions] to the end that all are related and combined into an effective unit capable of being directed toward accomplishment of common goals."

It is important that nurse-managers understand the functions to be performed by the staff prior to considering the physical factors or the personnel who will actually carry out the nursing care on the unit. Once established, the functions can be grouped with other functions to create positions that require physical factors. When the parameters of the functions are determined and the physical factors are established, then the requirements of personnel in a generic sense can be delineated. Then the search for appropriate personnel to fill the created positions can begin. This brief explanation represents an overview of what will be investigated in organizing in nursing.

In a hospital setting there are certain organic functions representing work performed that can be differentiated from other work. Thus, functions can be subsequently delineated into more discrete actions and activities. The organic functions of a hospital may be given as follows:

1. Physician care
2. Nursing care
3. Administrative and support functions

There are many ways in which organic functions can be determined, but for the purpose of this discussion, we will use the taxonomy of physician care, nursing care, and administration and support functions.

Nursing-care functions, determined in accordance with patient's needs, are (Eckelberry, 1975, p.75):

1 Giving supportive nursing care
2 Giving remedial, curative nursing care
3 Giving reeducative nursing care
4 Giving preventive nursing care

Eckelberry (1975, p. 75) further elaborates these functions into related activities as, for example, in the case of "giving preventive nursing care":

> Instructing patient before surgery how to breathe, cough, turn, and use a trapeze
> Demonstrating how to apply elastic bandages to aid venous circulation
> Teaching the pregnant woman relaxation exercises
> Helping parents learn developmental needs of infant during the first six to eight weeks of life
> Helping parents anticipate growth and developmental patterns of the preschooler
> Helping families prepare for progressive changes in long-term illness of a family member

These related activities can be subdivided further into specific subactivities (skills). Consider the first related activity: Instructing patient before surgery how to breathe, cough, turn and use a trapeze. We observe the subactivities to be performed before surgery as:

1. Teaching patient how to breathe
2. Teaching patient how to cough
3. Teaching patient how to turn
4. Teaching patient how to use a trapeze

The assumption without being overly basic at this stage is that certain knowledge and skills will be brought to the patient-care situation. The summary of this discussion is shown in Table 7-1.

You should realize that the organic functions used in this example are not to be considered a mutually exclusive set. Hence, these organic functions are not totally independent functions. There are major segments of each function that are independently ascertained and delivered. However, the degree of interface among all three organic functions must be seen.

The various levels of functions can be delineated to a basic motion. In some cases these refer to the turning and positioning of patients. In many hospital settings industrial engineers have studied the various activities on nursing units in hopes of establishing increased efficiency primarily in terms of economy of time performed and its concomitant anticipated reduction in staffing costs. In some cases enhancement of efficiency has been realized and costs contained. These types of studies have usually elicited negative reactions from nursing staff with expressed

Table 7-1 Functions—An Example

Organic Functions	(1) Nursing Functions
Physician care	Giving supportive nursing care
Nursing care (1)	Giving remedial, curative nursing care
Administrative and	Giving reeducative nursing care
support functions	Giving preventive nursing care (2)
(2) Giving Preventive Nursing Care	
	(3) Instructing patient before surgery
Instructing patient before surgery how	how to breathe, cough, turn, and use
to breathe, cough, turn, and use a	a trapeze
trapeze (3)	
	Before surgery
Demonstrating how to apply elastic	Teaching patient how to breathe
bandages to aid venous circulation	Teaching patient how to cough
Teaching pregnant woman relaxation	Teaching patient how to turn
exercises	Teaching patient how to use a trapeze
Helping parents learn developmental	
needs of infant during the first	
6 to 8 weeks of life	
Helping parents anticipate growth	
and developmental patterns of	
the preschooler	
Helping family prepare for progressive	
changes in long-term illness of	
family member	

Source: Adapted from Grace K. Eckelberry, *Administration of Comprehensive Nursing Care* (New York: Appleton-Century-Crofts, 1971), p. 75

concern over possible effects on the quality of patient care that may be delivered. In any event it is important that functions be defined and delineated in a manner that will permit the delivery of quality patient care with reasonable costs to the patient.

PRIMARY AND SECONDARY FUNCTIONS

In order to understand the organic functions in an organizational sense, it is necessary to determine which functions are primary and which functions are secondary. To do this in a hospital setting, we must look at the primary goals of the organization. As previously mentioned, one overriding goal of a hospital is to render quality patient care hopefully to secure the restoration of health of hospitalized patients. Thus, the central thrust of the hospital is to provide care through its organic functions of physician care and nursing care. Other functions performed in the organizational setting must be viewed as supportive and ancillary to the primary mission of the organization. These functions as defined earlier would comprise administration and support functions.

In terms of organizational theory, the functions that directly affect the accomplishment of the mission of the organization are considered to be primary functions of the organization. Since the primary function of the hospital is patient care, physician care and nursing care constitute the dual primary functions of the hospital. All other functions are then considered to be secondary. This differentiation should in no way be construed to imply that secondary or support functions are not important. However, the impact generated by these secondary functions on the primary mission is not as direct as those of physician care and nursing care.

To assist in the understanding of primary and secondary functions as they relate to the mission of the organization, consider the following examples. As mentioned, a nurse working in a hospital setting with a mission of delivering patient care is considered to be performing a primary function. However, a nurse who is hired to work for a school district, the primary mission of which is education, would be performing a secondary role in relation to the primary mission of the school. A third example would be the case of a nurse who is hired by the school district to teach health education classes. In this case, the nurse's role is primarily to teach; consequently, the nurse would be performing a primary function. Thus, it is important to relate the function performed with the primary mission of the organization to determine if the function is primary or secondary in nature.

FUNCTIONS AND ORGANIZATIONAL MATURATION

To develop a perspective of how functions are adapted and changed as an organization matures, consider the following situation. A primary-care physician has just finished a residency and is beginning a practice in a developing small community. At the outset of the practice, the physician's patient load is light but is expected to grow. The physician secures a loan from a local bank, rents office space, and purchases basic equipment for the office operations. A part-time receptionist is hired to do the scheduling of appointments and some typing. At this point in time, the organization of the office is as shown in Figure 7-1.

Soon the practice grows, the part-time help is full-time, and you are hired as the office nurse. The full-time clerical staff expands, and the receptionist is doing scheduling only and a full-time secretary/bookkeeper is hired. Now the organization of the office has changed as depicted in Figure 7-2.

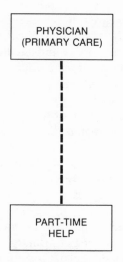

Figure 7-1 New Practice

The practice grows to a point where the physician feels that the patient load justifies a second physician; so a partnership is formed. The organization that had expanded vertically now expands horizontally as well. Thus, the organization now appears as in Figure 7-3.

The solid lines indicate primary functions of care performed in the

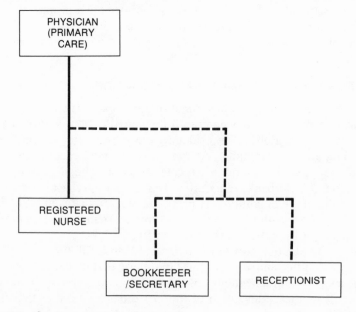

Figure 7-2 Practice—Vertically Expanded

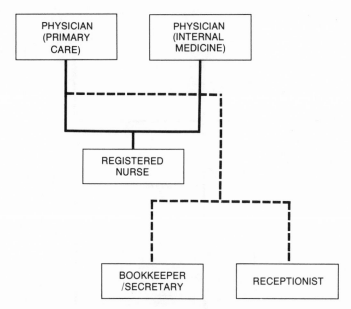

Figure 7-3 Practice—Horizontally Expanded

office. The dotted lines illustrate secondary or ancillary functions that support the primary functions as performed by the physicians and nurse.

As the practice expands and your work load increases, you request that a licensed practical (vocational) nurse be hired to assist you. The physicans concur with your request. Shortly thereafter, a third physician joins the partnership, and they ask you to coordinate nursing care. You now request a second LPN to assist. The practice has expanded and is organized as shown in Figure 7-4.

When the first licensed practical nurse was hired, you were faced with the problem of considering all the nursing functions that you had previously performed; the kinds of activities that could be legally performed by an LPN, and given the individual hired, how much work could be given to that individual. With the addition of the second LPN, what would constitute the best assignment of activities between the two LPNs now working in the office? You decide to assign one LPN to work with the obstetrician/gynecologist. The other LPN is assigned to work with the primary-care physician and the internist, with you functioning as a coordinator of nursing care and floating to relieve peaks in patient case loads.

What we have observed with the growth of this practice is a process of functionalization. This process consists of splitting the original function of providing *all* nursing care in the practice into components. The components were determined by examining the activities and assigning those activities that were legally assignable, given the education and

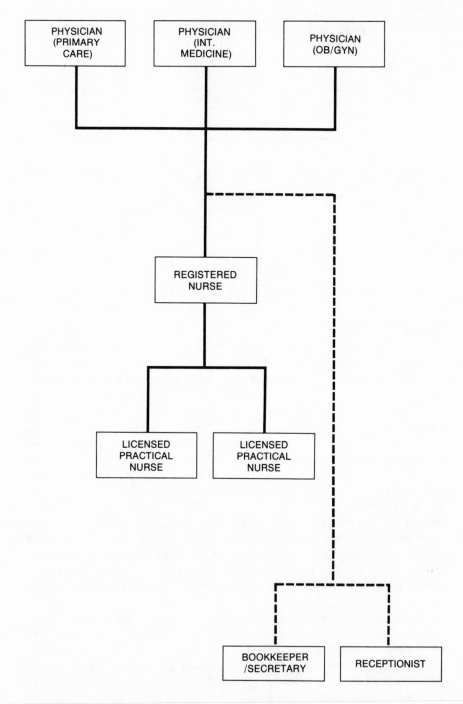

Figure 7-4 Practice Augmented by LPNs—Expanded Further (Vertically)

experience of the new employees. Throughout the decision-making process, you took into consideration the nature and extent of the differences and similarities of the practices of the three physicians and the direct implications of differences and similarities of nursing care that would be required.

Over the next few years the practice expands and additional physicians are brought into the practice. Additional registered nurses and licensed practical nurses are hired. The physicians feel that to ensure the provision nursing care at a level commensurate with standards, you should continue as coordinator of nursing care. As the practice expands it becomes apparent that your role of coordinator is becoming more and more difficult to accomplish. Finally, you come to the conclusion that you cannot handle the coordination of that many nurses. Let us examine the organization at this time to ascertain the problem. (see Figure 7-5).

The problem is clearly noted that you as nurse-coordinator have too many people to coordinate. You are, in fact, unable to coordinate properly or to control what is happening. Thus, the span of control is too great. Span of control refers to the number of individuals who report directly to you as a supervisor.

The original work on span of control was done by Hamilton, Graicunas, and Urwick. Sir Ian Hamilton (1921, p.229) suggested that there should be a specific span limit placed on the number of individuals reporting to a manager. This span was established at three to six persons. Later, V. A. Graicunas (1937,pp.183–184) developed a mathematical relationship that supported Hamilton's suggestion of an upper limit of six persons.

In establishing any span of control in an organization, nurse-managers must consider the complexity of the work to be accomplished and the capacity of the individuals performing those roles. The extremes of this situation are demonstrated by the complex situation with individuals who need constant supervision. In this case the span of control should be limited (shortened) to perhaps two to three individuals. When the work is not complex and done by well-qualified individuals, the limit could be raised above the two to three as suggested by the previous case. When nurse-managers are faced with a span-of-control situation, professional judgement must be used in establishing the appropriate number of employees reporting to a supervisor. Urwick (1933, p. 8) probably best summarized the work of Graicunas on span of control, "No superior can supervise directly the work of more than five, or at the most, six individuals whose work interlocks."

PROBLEM OF FUNCTIONAL BALANCE

In discussing the problem of balance, Koontz (1966) states that "it can readily be seen that the span of management problems, like most in life,

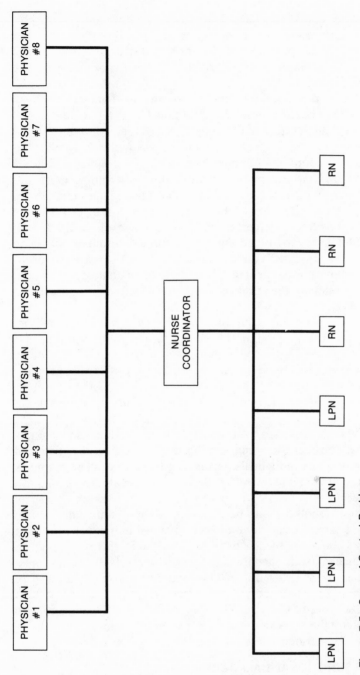

Figure 7-5 Span-of-Control Problem

raises a difficult question of balance. In general, the narrower the span, the more complete the supervision can be, although there are many cases of narrow spans where the superior, having too little to do, tends to oversupervise his subordinates.'' The problem of functional balance is interrelated to the problem of span of control. As we observed from the example in this chapter, the functions of the organization will be initially differentiated vertically and horizontally. As the organization grows and becomes more complex with increased patient load, such splitting of functions is logical and necessary. If too much functionalization has occured, the organization may incur unnecessary costs and personnel. Likewise, too little functionalization can result in overtaxing individuals and a possible decrease in effectiveness. Inherent in the extent of differentiation is the establishment of appropriate levels of supervision over the various functions that have been delineated. The greater the differentiation and the greater the span of control, the less the organization has grown vertically. In general, then, the less the differentiation and the less the span of control, the more the organization has grown vertically.

Herbert Simon (1947, pp.26–27) observed the problem facing the manager in examining the concept of functional balance and span of control:

> A contradictory proverb of administration can be stated which, though it is not so familiar as the principle of span of control, can be supported by arguments of equal plausibility. The proverb in question is the following: "Administrative efficiency is enhanced by keeping at a minimum the number of organizational levels through which a matter must pass before it is acted on." In many situations the results to which this principle leads are in direct contradiction to the requirements of the span of control.

Thus, we see the great importance of the delicate balance that must be maintained in the organization. Certainly an organization should attempt to reduce the number or organizational levels to improve communications, but it should not be carried to a point that would hamper reasonable limits of span of control. It must be realized that the limits of span of control are very real and cannot be ignored in the decision-making process of functionalization. Hence, the balancing act of the manager in functionalization of the organization is to trade inefficient organization levels with the real need of a good span of control.

SUMMARY

A frequent problem on the nursing units is one of organization. Many of these problems stem from the fact that the basic foundation of organization or unit have not been effectively accomplished, and as a result, we see the aberrations of the basic foundation. Before the organizational aspects of a nursing unit can be examined, it is necessary that functions to be performed in the unit be developed. This means that the functions should be determined prior to managerial decision making with regard to physical factors or personnel. Once functions have been established, they can be grouped with other functions to create position descriptions. Likewise, physical factors coupled with parameters of functions will set the stage for generic personnel requirements.

We examined a hospital setting with three organic functions: physician care, nursing care, and administration and support functions. Nursing care as an organic function was then subdivided into functions of nursing care. We then elaborated one of these functions into related activities, which was then divided into discrete subactivities. The resulting subactivities reflect delineation to a level of basic motions.

We noted that the organic functions are not totally independent. Major segments of each organic function are independently ascertained, but a certain degree of interface exists among all three functions.

The case of determining where organic functions are primary or secondary functions was reviewed. The key to making such a determination rests with the role relationship of the organic functions to the primary goals of the organization. In the hospital setting where the rendering of quality patient care is the primary goal, the organic functions of physician care and nursing care must be considered as primary functions. Administration and support functions are considered to be of a secondary nature. We further elaborated that secondary functions should not be considered unimportant.

We used a case of a physician's developing practice to demonstrate that as the organization matures, it will differentiate functions and grow both vertically and horizontally. Focusing on the role of a registered nurse, we examined the process of functionalization. Functionalization consists of splitting the functions into components to be performed by others. The coordinating role of the nurse was carried to a point where the span of control exceeded reasonable limits. Span of control is a concept that refers to the number of individuals who report directly to a manager.

We reviewed the work of Hamilton and Graicunas, which established limits for span of control ranging from three to six. A further examination of this concept revealed that nurse-managers must consider the complexity of the work to be accomplished and the capacity of individuals supporting that work activity.

Finally, we considered the problem of functional balance. The relationship of functional balance and span of control as interrelated brought to a focus the key to the functions and management in nursing. The greater the differentiation and the span of control, the less the organization has grown vertically. The less differentiation and span of control, the more the organization has grown vertically. The problem nurse-managers face is the proper balance of functionalization and span of control. These two concepts tend to work in opposition to each other. Certainly administrative efficiency is better with few organizational levels, but this appears to be in contradiction with a reasonable span of control. The balance of these two concepts is imperative to enhancing coordination, control, and communication in the organization and the resulting delivery of quality patient care.

BIBLIOGRAPHY

Eckelberry, Grace K. *Administration of Comprehensive Nursing Care.* New York: Appleton-Century-Crofts, 1971.

Flippo, Edwin B. *Management: A Behavioral Approach,* 2nd ed. Boston: Allyn & Bacon, 1970.

Graicunas, V. A. "Relationship in Organization." In *Papers on the Science of Administration,* edited by L. Gulick and L. Urwick. New York: Institute of Public Administration, Columbia University, 1937.

Hamilton, Sir Ian. *The Soul and Body of an Army.* London: Edward Arnold, 1921.

Koontz, Harold. "Making Theory Operational: The Span of Management." *The Journal of Management Studies;* vol. 3, no. 3 (October 1966): 229–243.

Simon, Herbert A. *Administrative Behavior.* New York: Macmillan, 1947.

Urwick, Lyndall F. *Scientific Principles and Organization.* New York: American Management Association, Institute of Management Series no. 19, 1938.

Chapter 8

The Organizing Process in Nursing

The structure of organizations is probably the most thoroughly studied area of management. Organizational theorists and managers who have worked extensively in the operational environment agree that an organizational structure cannot be allowed just to evolve. Organizations that have merely evolved without proper planning and strategy are confused, disordered, overstaffed, and perform poorly. Before establishing an organizational structure, it is necessary that the basic components (functions and activities) be delineated. These activities will be incorporated in the final organizational structure in such a way that functional balance and resources can be deployed appropriately to permit the organization to meet its objectives.

Chandler (1962) provided the foundational basis of the fact that the strategy of organizing must precede the development of the actual structure itself. Organizational structure provides the framework for the attainment of organizational missions including goals and objectives. Since activities support functions and objectives, it is obvious that work with objectives and strategy must precede expenditure of time on organizational structure. In other words, we cannot conceive of constructing a building from the top floor down.

In the previous chapter we examined activities that might be performed by a nurse on a unit. We noted that these activities could be grouped into functions of nursing. At this point we will develop concepts of design of jobs that are based on activities and are conceived on a task-focused basis. Later we will see that the actual assignment of individuals to those developed positions should be accomplished through a congruence of fit. In all the planning and organizing, we should never lose sight of the fact that the job itself is performed by the individual so assigned by the nurse-manager.

CONCEPTS OF DESIGN

As nurse-managers examine the various functions to be performed, there are many ways in which the design of positions may be accomplished. These functions as previously mentioned were developed from the objectives of the organization. With these facts in mind, managers could decide to group functions that are similar in nature and that tend to support similar objectives. This approach is used in the development of various departments and units in many health-care settings. In an overall sense of patient-care delivery, this approach has merit and has demonstrated increased quality of care as evidenced by decreased mortality rates in many units. This development can be illustrated in the establishment of critical-care units, including such units as coronary-care and neonatal intensive-care units.

In a similar fashion within some nursing units, positions have been developed that provide for a very narrow position role whereby a series of nurses provide specialized tasks for an individual patient. An example of this approach would be the position description for a nurse whose sole responsibility consisted of "passing medications." This type of approach would seem to support the concept of volume that is a prerequisite to specialization. Likewise, specialization can lead to certain economies in many organizational settings, but it does not necessarily appear to be true in a health-care organization. With increased specialization in a total sense patient-care cost has usually increased. It is absolutely essential in considering specialization that sufficient volume of work exists to maintain quality care.

Behavioral scientists have attacked the design of positions along this line of repetition of similar tasks. A primary drawback is the lack of consideration of existing personnel with various interests and capabilities. Obviously, both views should not be accepted. A balance of both approaches would appear reasonable. Perhaps the best approach considers both aspects with functions being formulated on a framework basis followed by the goodness of fit of the individual. In establishing the design of positions, it is important to watch for gaps and overlaps. Certainly the designer must be assured that all tasks have been assigned to positions, and care should be taken to minimize unnecessary duplication on assignment of tasks.

As you will recall, the organization identified its mission, which was subsequently identified as a series of goals, and later delineated further as functions and activities. Following this logical sequence of events, the designer of positions must look at a matrix of various functions to be performed, and using the previously developed concepts of design, assign functions to the various positions. The approach to design is interrelated and dependent to a great extent on the philosophy of the organization with respect to the pattern of delivery of nursing care. Various philosophies will be covered in the following chapter on organizational structure.

Regardless of the philosophy of delivery, it is necessary that nurse-managers secure an understanding of the categories and roles of nursing personnel that can be used in a unit. In addition, the nurse-manager must be thoroughly familiar with management concepts of responsibility, authority, and accountability.

PERSONNEL RESOURCES

There are many categories of nursing personnel in the United States. The variations in nurse-practice acts and the proliferation of position descriptions preclude a definition of services that may be rendered. However, some *generalized* categories of personnel resources can be considered.

Nurses' aides usually have a few weeks of formal training. They administer hygienic care and in some health-care settings take vital signs and record fluid intake and output. Aides perform their duties under the supervision of a registered nurse or physician.

Licensed practical nurses or vocational nurses have completed a course of study through a vocational school or community college. The LPN renders nursing care to patients with relatively simple nursing problems. In all cases such care is provided under the supervision of a registered nurse or physician.

Registered nurses are licensed to practice nursing in a variety of health-care settings. The RN is able to function with some degree of independence as a provider of primary nursing care. The principal programs that prepare RNs for license to practice are the associate degree program, the diploma program, and the bachelor's degree program. Most recently the expanded role of the registered nurse has evolved that has been identified as the nurse practitioner. The ANA has worked to define this expanded role; however, a general consensus has not been reached.

In terms of personnel use, it is helpful to examine the roles that may be considered by graduates that lead to eligibility for state licensing as RNS. The Western Council on Higher Education for Nursing (1967) concluded that the associate degree graduates are able to function with some autonomy as providers of primary nursing care. Their educational preparation did not provide sufficient background for management responsibilities in nursing units.

Graduates of hospital diploma programs can function as nurse generalists in acute-care settings and can provide nursing care through therapeutic rehabilitative and preventive regimens to patients and groups of patients (National League for Nursing, 1971).

The bachelor's degree graduates function as providers of direct patient care, as teachers, as leader-supervisors of members of health groups, as collaborators and effective members of health teams, as interpreters of nursing activities to allied professionals in developing plans for optimal health programs, as assistants in research, as representatives of nursing to outside groups, and as inquiring persons (WCHEN, 1968).

Alutto, Hrebiniak, and Alonso (1971) found that in spite of educational differences and any initial personality differences or similarities that graduates of all three RN programs did not differ in terms of cognitive commitment to professional nursing, employing organizations, and clinical specialties. Research by Highriter (1969) and Davis (1974) indicates that differences in education may affect behavior.

Trends in nursing roles have been occurring to a great extent during the 1960s and 1970s. Consequently, we have observed the evolution of the clinical nurse specialist, nurse clinician, and nurse practitioner. Uniformity of definition and role of these nursing activities has not been finalized. However, it is necessary that the current thinking about these roles be discussed.

Generally, the clinical nurse specialist will have a master's degree with education in a specialty. The primary objective of this specialist is to counter the trend of moving the nurse away from bedside nursing. The return of the nurse to the bedside is to direct patient care and to provide greater comprehensiveness, continuity, and coordination of patient services. The clinical nurse specialist will function as a partner with the physician in the unit (Brown, 1971).

The nurse clinician functions as a generalist and is usually employed at a middle-level position of practice because of demonstrated advanced clinical competence. Academic preparation is that of any RN program.

The expanded role of nurse practitioner is one that primarily functions in an ambulatory setting. In addition to entry from any RN program, the nurse practitioner usually has an additional apprenticeship that may last as long as one year. In most cases (Murray, 1973) the nurse will work closely with a physician, although some practitioners have been practicing on an independent basis.

It certainly would appear that the role of the nurse is unclear. The direction of change is quite clear; the role of the nurse will expand over time. Adaptability to future developments would seem to be best anticipated through the interaction model recommended by the National Commission for the Study of Nursing and Nursing Education (Lysaught, 1970). This dynamic model of nurse/physician interaction is based on patient needs and provides for nursing assessment, intervention, and instruction for patients dependent on patient condition and environmental factors.

Much work has gone on and will continue to differentiate roles where feasible. The programs in general emphasize technical competency and skill as well as problem-solving and using nursing judgement. Graduates of RN and LPN programs in the operational environment of a health-care setting are many times expected to assume the role of the nurse manager for which they have had little formal education. Didactic preparation in nursing management as well as a management practicum is necessary. Nurse-managers must bring management knowledge and expertise to the unit to ensure the effective use of resources and delivery of quality nursing care.

In contemplating the roles that may be performed by various nursing personnel, you must remember that functions are limited in almost all cases by the nurse practice act of your state. In the case of your particular nursing unit, many nursing activities and their assignment must be accomplished in conformance with your hospital policy as provided by your organization policy manual.

TOOLS OF THE NURSE-MANAGER

The nurse-manager has three management tools that must be used with care and thoughtfulness. These tools are responsibility, authority, and accountability. As goals lead to objectives and objectives to functions, so functions lead to responsibility. In this discussion responsibility will refer to the obligation of the nurse to carry out work or functions. The nurse-manager is the principal source for delegating responsibility to other nursing personnel. This responsibility for delegation has been passed on to the nurse-manager by the next higher level in the organization. Thus, we see that responsibility represents a series of obligations established between various levels of the organization. You must remember that when you delegate responsibility, you cannot relieve yourself of the original responsibility. Therefore, when you delegate responsibility you are permitting someone else to perform functions that you were assigned by your manager.

In nursing units, staff is held responsible for certain functions. However, these functions cannot be performed as intended because the nurse-manager has not provided sufficient authority to carry out the assigned responsibility. Authority is a right to decide, command, and perform the assigned responsibility. The need for clear authority is a precondition to make responsibility acceptable (Drucker, 1973, p. 272). There is a need to ensure a parity of responsibility and authority. Without parity, a nurse cannot function effectively in the delivery of quality nursing care. Thus, authority is a permission to proceed with the assignment (Newman, Simmer & Warren, 1967, p. 84), with transferred rights to direct the work of other people and to use equipment and supplies in the unit. For example, as a manager of a new graduate nurse, you may wish to provide responsibility that is greater than delegated authority. Jucius (1967, p. 80) has suggested that as a new employee acquires skills and the manager's trust, the amount of authority can be increased to a level of parity with responsibility.

Once nursing personnel have been given responsibility with a parity of authority, then it is appropriate to hold them accountable for performance. If, as a nurse-manager, you have not provided parity of responsibility and authority, it is unjust to hold staff accountable for performance. In an organizational design sense, it is important that the concept of single accountability be implemented as much as possible. Nursing personnel should only be accountable to one manager. This approach usually results in better coordination and understanding of role expectations. Implicit with single accountability is unity of command for each employee assigned to a nursing unit. As an organization grows and becomes more complex it is more difficult to maintain single accountability. However, unity of command can be maintained in spite of increasing complexity of organization. Next we will consider the structure of organizations in nursing.

SUMMARY

Before establishing an organizational structure, it is necessary to delineate basic components. Strategy must precede the development of the structure. We examined various concepts of design. Designs should establish the grouping of functions based on the objectives of the organization. Specialization within health care and delivery of nursing care was included as a design consideration. In examining specialization we noted that sufficient volume is a precondition to maintaining quality of care. The approach to design is interrelated and dependent to a great extent on the philosophy of the organization with respect to the pattern of delivery of nursing care.

In designing positions it is necessary that the nurse-manager secure an understanding of the categories and roles of nursing personnel to be used on a unit. The educational backgrounds of nurses' aides, LPNs, and RNs were reviewed. We noted that major trends in nursing roles have occurred during the 1960s and 1970s. These trends have resulted in new roles for nurses, such as clinical nurse specialists, nurse clinicians, and nurse practitioners. A definitive future role of these positions is not totally clear. However, the direction of change is quite evident—the role of the nurse will expand. Adaptability to these changing roles is probably best anticipated by using the interactive model recommended by the National Commission for the Study of Nursing and Nursing Education. All nursing roles to be performed on the unit must be accomplished in compliance with nurse practice acts and local hospital policy.

The nurse-manager has three management tools that must be used with care and thoughtfulness: responsibility, authority, and accountability. The concept of parity of responsibility and authority provided a necessary and sufficient condition to require accountability from employees on the unit. It was recommended that single accountability and unity of command concepts be used in the organizing process to enhance coordination and understanding of role expectations.

BIBLIOGRAPHY

Alutto, Joseph A.; Hrebiniak, Lawrence; and Alonso, Ramon. "A Study of Differential Socialization for Members of One Professional Occupation." *Journal of Health and Social Behavior* 12 (1971): 140–147.

Barrett, Jean. "The Nurse Specialist Practitioner: A Study." *Nursing Outlook,* vol. 20, no. 8 (1972): 524–527.

Brown, Esther Lucille. *Nursing Reconsidered: A Study of Change,* Parts 1 and 2. Philadelphia: J. B. Lippincott, 1971.

Chandler, Alfred D. *Strategy and Structure.* Cambridge, Mass.: M.I.T. Press, 1962.

Davis, B. G. "The Effects of Heads of Nursing Education on Patient Care: A Replication." *Nursing Research* 23 (March–April 1974): 150–155.

Drucker, Peter F. *Management: Tasks, Responsibilities, and Practices.* New York: Harper & Row, 1973.

Georgopoulos, Basil, and Christman, Luther. "The Clinical Nurse Specialist: A Role Model." *American Journal of Nursing,* vol. 70, no. 1030 (May 1970): 1030–1039.

Highriter, M. E. "Nurse Characteristics and Patient Progress." *Nursing Research* 18 (December 1969): 484–500.

Jucius, Michael J. *Personnel Management,* 6th ed. Homewood, Ill.: Irwin, 1967.

Little D. "The Nurse Specialist." *American Journal of Nursing* 67 (1967): 552.

Lysaught, Jerome P. *An Abstract for Action.* New York: McGraw-Hill, 1970.

Murray, Raymond H., and Ross, Shirley A. "Training the Nurse Practitioner." *Hospitals* 47 (1973): 93.

National League for Nursing Council of Diploma Programs, May 1971.

Newman, William H.; Simmer, Charles; and Warren, E. Kirby. *The Process of Management: Concepts, Behavior and Practice,* 2nd ed. Englewood Cliffs, N.J.: Prentice-Hall, 1967.

Simms,L. L. "The Clinical Nurse Specialist: An Experiment." *Nursing Outlook,* vol. 13, no. 8 (August 1965): 26–28.

Western Council on Higher Education for Nursing, Baccalaureate Degree Seminar, April, 1968.

Western Council on Higher Education for Nursing, Curriculum Content Committee of the Association Degree Seminar, 1967.

Chapter 9

Structure of Organizations in Nursing

To complete our formal organizing process in nursing we will now examine the various structures that can be established. As a nurse works in different units and in various hospitals, it becomes quite apparent that there are many ways to deliver nursing care throughout the nation. Certainly different delivery systems have shown varying degrees of effectiveness. It is difficult, at best, to say that one delivery system has been consistently better than another system. This situation is primarily due to the differences in dependent variables. Some of these variables include patient needs, setting, abilities of nursing staff, abilities of the medical staff, extent and effectiveness of administrative support, the nursing philosophy, and the effectiveness of ancillary functions in the hospital.

STRUCTURAL DELIVERY SYSTEMS

In actual practice nurse-managers have some degree of influence on many of these dependent variables. One variable on which the nurse-manager may have the greatest impact over time is the nursing philosophy of the hospital. The philosophy may be expressed in basic delivery systems of nursing care.

The first and probably oldest system of delivery is the case method. This system is used when the philosophy dictates that a single nurse is assigned to a single patient. Such an assignment is predicated on the need for continuous care and observation for a definite period of time. This system emphasizes the wholistic approach to patient care. In other words, the nurse is responsible for total nursing care of the assigned patient. Today, this philosophy and approach to nursing care delivery can be seen most often in the care of the critically ill patient in critical-care units. This approach is also used by private-duty nurses. From an education standpoint, the case method has been used for many years as the principal vehicle in assigning student nurses to patients (See Figure 9-1).

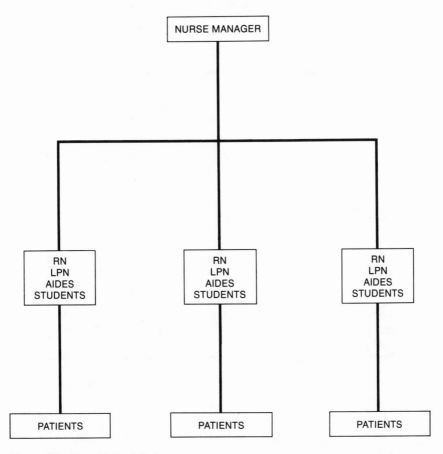

Figure 9-1 Case Method System

The second system involves the use of functions as the primary factor in the allocation of work and the assignment of personnel. Under this system the nurse is assigned to preset designed functions such as only passing medications or only administering treatments. This approach is task-oriented. These functional systems are couched in a mass production mold, generally permit a conservation of manpower, and are usually favored by administration. This system is widely used throughout the nation. Rationale for such extensive use was the shortage of nursing personnel and apparent cost-containment aspects. Consideration of other systems has resulted from nursing staff dissatisfaction of the functional system, as well as research that has questioned its cost effectiveness (See Figure 9-2).

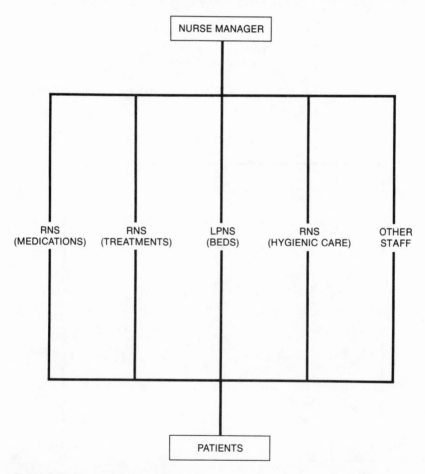

Figure 9-2 Functional Method System

The third system, known as the team method, evolved primarily as a result of World War II and its impact on the health-care system. During that time a tremendous expansion of the armed forces drew many nurses out of the civilian health-care sector. Consequently, civilian hospitals were extremely short of nursing staff. Concurrent advances in medical technology resulted in the development of new medical technicians and specialists in the hospital setting. During this time health-care delivery experienced new drugs, treatment plans, complex equipment, and a virtual explosion of new knowledge for medical practice. Consequently, the nurse and patient unit became the focus of this new complexity.

Under the team method the professional nurse acts as a manager to facilitate the work of a group of health personnel to meet the health needs of patients in a unit. This approach considers the concept of accomplishing group responsibilities through a team process whereby the nurse team leader plans, organizes, directs, and controls the care provided by the team. The care delivered through a group delivery concept has a primary focus of individualized health care. The foundational basis of the team method is not a new concept and is grounded in philosophy. The team approach to problem-solving is quite common in many situations. Coordination and communication effectiveness are essential conditions to the success of the team method (see Figure 9-3).

The fourth and newest system of nursing-care delivery is primary care. This concept was developed in the late 1960s. Primary care envisions the direct nurse-to-patient relationship. Under this system the nurse has total responsibility for planning and directing patient care for 24 hours a day for the duration of patient need for care. This system requires that the nurse assigned to that patient provide a comprehensive care plan with concomitant directions for other personnel to carry out and continue the planned care. In this role the primary nurse coordinates with other nurses, physicians, and ancillary personnel. Continuity of care can be a positive aspect of this system due to the specific assignment of responsibility and accountability (see Figure 9-4).

Certainly each system has definite advantages and disadvantages depending on the situation and the relative strengths of the dependent variables. Each system creates a linking of components and functions so that structure permits the organization to take shape. The structural connections all have common elements that include the management tools previously discussed—namely, responsibility, authority, and accountability.

From an organizational standpoint, the case-method system and the primary-care system provide the greatest direct access of the RN to the patient. These two methods stress the wholistic approach to patient care and thus provide the best opportunity for continuity of care and responsiveness of staff to changing conditions of patients. Certainly, these ap-

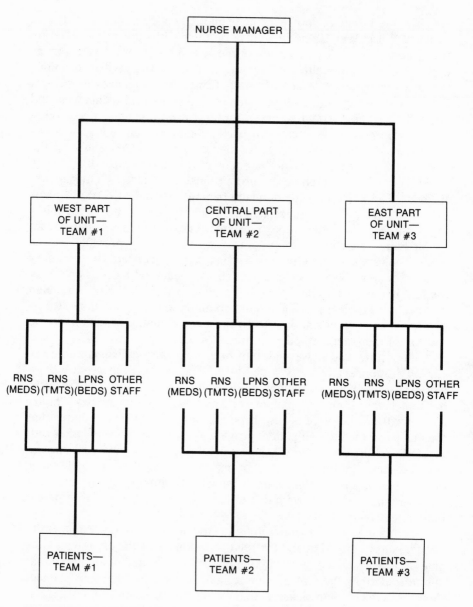

Figure 9-3 Team Method System

parent advantages can be substantially offset if the span of control of the nurse is so wide that immediate responsiveness to changed conditions has been precluded.

The other two systems are not wholistic and do not generally allow for as great a direct access and as quick a response time as do the other

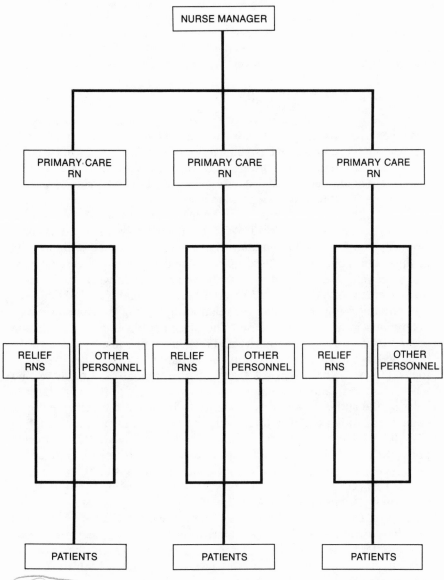

Figure 9-4 Primary-Care Method System

two methods. Both methods use somewhat the same approach but differ because the team approach usually uses a smaller territorial area for assignment versus the entire unit for the functional method. Thus, the team system may be viewed as a smaller version of the functional method.

It must be clearly understood that the four systems as presented are for the purpose of demonstrating basic differences in models of delivery.

In actual practice many variations exist as nurse-managers establish innovative approaches that better fit their own situations, patient needs,
and responsibilities. Detailed coverage of implications for communication
and coordination of these methods will be discussed later.

STRUCTURAL CONSIDERATIONS

Given the four structural delivery systems, it is necessary to consider
some generic aspects of structures that may be developed. First, nurse-
managers undertake an extensive analysis of decisions that will be made
in the future. In thinking through the objectives to be accomplished,
managers should decide what decisions are likely to be made to ensure
adequate performance and the accomplishment of objectives, more specifically, what kind of decisions are to be made and at what organizational
level should they be effectuated. Who should be involved in the decisions,
who will be affected by them, and who should be informed of the results
of those decisions? Once these questions have been addressed and answers secured, the decision locators made and certain work established,
the placement of authority and responsibility is a reality.

Next, it is imperative that the relationship among the components be
determined in a structural sense. The placement of components in the
organization given their authority and responsibility must be finalized. In
other words, nurse-managers should ascertain with what other managers
they will work, what affect will these other operations have on them, and
what affect their unit operations will have on other operations. In considering the authority and responsibility to be given, the placement of a
component within the structure should be designed in such a manner so
that the number of working relationships is minimized. In this design
phase the essential interrelationships to the accomplishment of objectives
must incorporate features that permit immediate accessibility to key decision makers in the management process. Thus, a need should exist for
each interrelationship that would directly enhance the accomplishment of
objectives. Confusion can often exist in the design phase between where
decisions are made and how they interrelate. Usually the interrelatedness
aspect determines design flow of decisions, and as a result, the interrelationship analysis should take precedence over the initial analysis of decision locators.

DIAGNOSING STRUCTURAL PROBLEMS

From the outset, it must be stated that no organization has been designed
and developed that can be considered the "best." Organization design of
components and structure is an ongoing activity. Changes occur inside
and outside the organization that can redesign the operations. Regardless

of the source of change, it is important that changes be improvements toward accomplishing objectives and not merely changes for the sake of change. Nurse-managers must maintain a constant vigil to watch for symptoms that can result in decreased organizational effectiveness.

These symptoms can manifest themselves in various ways. We have stressed the need to minimize the number of working relationships. An organization will often develop more levels of management, which produces a situation whereby the chain of command has been lengthened and responsiveness and effectiveness have been hampered. It is important that the chain of command be kept as short as possible to preclude the occurrence of this problem. Corrective action for this problem usually constrains the increases in levels of management.

Another common indication of organizational problems is when the institution undergoes continuous reorganization. Such a case is the classic one of change for the sake of change, and it usually results from the original design not having been properly thought through. Consequently, the organization is continuously trying to patch up problem areas that later manifest themselves in the same area or other areas. It is far better to do an in-depth extensive reevaluation of the entire structure and its inter-relationships and make one major reorganization, if organizational insta-bility appears to be of a chronic nature.

Other problems that surface quite frequently are evidenced by con-tinuous concern over the feelings of individuals and an extensive number of conferences to coordinate activities. This problem does not mean that the nurse-managers are not concerned with the individual nurses and with the needs of individuals as previously discussed. But rather, the design problem usually has resulted from overstaffing. The symptoms manifest themselves through friction, excessive arguments, and a general feeling of worrying about hurting someone's feelings. As a result, work is created to keep people busy. Needless to say, this type of work is not productive.

When the nurse-manager spends more time in conference, it is symptomatic of an organizational problem. The fundamental problem usually results from the fact that individuals' responsibilities have not been adequately defined, that the design of positions are too narrow, and that there is sufficient accessibility to the chain of command. Every effort should be made to minimize the need for conferences and to minimize the number of individuals who should attend such conferences.

SUMMARY

This chapter examined the structure of organizations in nursing. Many different nursing-care systems in the United States. Differences in de-pendent variables were noted as reasons for various levels of effectiveness in nursing care delivery. We examined the philosophy of nursing as expressed through structural delivery systems, and we reviewed the delivery systems, including the case-method system, functional-method system, team-method system, and primary-care system. The general characteristics of each system were covered. Some advantages and disadvantages of these systems were considered as they related to use of personnel and nurse accessibility to patients. We noted that the four models of delivery were used to demonstrate basic differences in delivery, and in actual nursing practice many modifications of these models will be experienced.

Structural considerations were given that included what, what kind, and at what management levels decisions should be made. In addition, the decisions regarding the interrelationship of components and their placement were examined. Confusion can often exist in this design phase of organization structures between where decisions are made and how they interrelate. We suggested that interrelatedness of design reflects the flow of decisions, and as a result, the interrelationship analysis should take precedent over the initial analysis of decision locators.

No organization has been designed and developed that can be considered as the best. However, some common structural problems can be identified and corrected through appropriate managerial action. Some common problems included increasing the levels of management, condition of continuous reorganization, continuous concern over the feelings of individuals, and an extensive number of conferences to coordinate activities. The vast majority of these problems can be alleviated by keeping the number of working relationships to a minimum, maintaining the shortest chain of command, clearly defining responsibilities, and by minimizing the number of conferences and the number of individuals attending these conferences.

BIBLIOGRAPHY

Aydelotte, M. "Standard I: Staffing for Quality Care." *Journal of Nursing Administration* (March–April 1973): 33–36.

Douglass, L. M. *Review of Team Nursing*. St. Louis: C. V. Mosby, 1973.

Drucker, Peter F. *Management: Tasks, Responsibilities, and Practices*. New York: Harper & Row, 1973.

Durbin, Richard L., and Springall, W. Herbert. *Organization and Administration of Health Care*. St. Louis: C. V. Mosby, 1969.

Hower, Ralph M., and Lorsch, Jay W. "Organizational Inputs" In *Systems Analysis in Organizational Behavior,* edited by John A. Seiler. Homewood, Ill. Richard D. Irwin and The Dorsey Press, 1967.

Kast, Fremont, and Rosenzweig, James E. *Organization and Management: A Systems Approach*. New York: McGraw-Hill, 1970.

Korn, Thora. *Nursing Team Leadership,* 2nd ed. Philadelphia: Saunders, 1966.

Manthey, M. "Primary Care Is Alive and Well in the Hospital." *American Journal of Nursing* 73 (1973): 83–87.

_____ et al. "Primary Nursing." *Nursing Forum* 9 (1970): 65–83.

Miller, D. I. "Standard II: Organization Is a Process." *Journal of Nursing Administration* (March–April 1972): 19–24.

Mott, Paul E. *The Characteristics of Effective Organizations.* New York: Harper & Row, 1972.

Norris, C. M. "Direct Access to the Patient." *American Journal of Nursing* 70 (1970): 1006–1010.

Pfiffner, John M., and Sherwood, Frank P. *Administrative Organization.* Englewood Cliffs, N.J.: Prentice-Hall, 1960.

Schulz, Rockwell, and Johnson, Alton C. *Management of Hospitals.* New York: McGraw-Hill, 1976.

Behavioral Influences on Organizing

Chapter 10

Informal Aspects of Organizations

In the earlier chapters of Part Three functions in nursing, the organizing process, and the structure of organizations in nursing were discussed. They have provided the foundation for the formal organization in nursing. We examined the structure and concepts of design, which were primarily task-oriented. However, as we all know, the assignments made on a nursing unit must fit both the needs of the situation and the needs of the individual. Hence, a goodness of fit must be secured to effectuate the sound management of the unit and the delivery of quality nursing care.

Certainly, the initial fit must come from a well-designed position and an individual who meets the specifications of the position. Thus, an a priori condition is necessary to a successful relationship but not sufficient to meet all of the needs of the individual. There are other needs that can be met through the working environment.

INFORMAL GROUPS

The organizational structure considered so far has been primarily an abstract entity. The composition of this structure has been that of jobs and not the people who will fill those jobs and make things happen. At this point, we observe the convergence of two aspects of organizations—on one hand the organizational structure as a formalized set of jobs and on the other hand the development of the group as a set of individuals.

As soon as individuals are introduced to the organizational setting, they constitute a formal work group. Simultaneously, these individuals interact with other individuals within and without their formal work groups. Thus, these informal groups are formed through a process of carrying out their assignments in the formal structure.

The relative size of the informal group depends on many factors, including physical proximity, number of continuous contacts, binding issues, and the needs of the individual. Berelson and Steiner (1964, p. 325) have defined the concept of groups as follows:

> By this term is meant an aggregate of people, from two up to an unspecified but not too large number, who associate together in face-to-face relationship over an extended period of time, who differentiate themselves in some regard from others around them, who are mutually aware of their membership in the group, and whose personnel relations are taken as an end in itself. It is impossible to specify a strict upper limit on the size of the informal group, except for the limitation imposed by the requirement that all the members be able to engage in direct personal relations at one time—which means, roughly, an upper limit of around fifteen to twenty. If the aggregate gets much larger than that, it begins to lose some of the quality of a small group or, indeed, begins to break up into small subgroups.

Homans (1950) provides some insight into the understanding of how groups form, interrelate, and become more cohesive. The theoretical construct he developed provides a taxonomy of "activity, interaction and sentiment" (p. 43). Basically the more activities people share, the more they interact, producing tangential results of sharing as well. The more they interact, the more they share and the more their sentiments tend to be shared. The extent of shared activities, compounded interactions, and increased sentiments can lead to group relationships totally external to the originating source of the group's formation.

The informal group developed from activities related to job performance that had not been formally prescribed by the formal organization. In other words, informal group activity constitutes those activities not officially sanctioned in any organization policy or manual.

The development of informal groups is a natural aberration of the formal organizational structure in a nursing unit. When nurse-managers bring individuals together in a unit, it is expected that they will communicate and work together. Managers assign certain duties and responsibilities to the nursing staff as part of their jobs. From that point, they proceed to execute their assignments and thereby interact with other personnel. However, it is through this process that many unintended consequences occur. Individuals on the unit will express opinions about their formal organization and how it is being managed. This situation develops to a point whereby an entire communications network has been developed that can exclude management. The informal communication network is usually referred to as "the grapevine." Depending on the construction of this network, personnel on the unit can become aware of situations prior to the nurse-manager's hearing about it through formal channels of communication. However, astute nurse-managers can use this informal channel of communication if they are aware of its existence and if they use it with sensitivity. The more nurse-managers work to keep personnel on the unit informed of current developments, the less likely will be the need for extensive communication through this informal network.

RATIONALE FOR INFORMAL GROUPS

Informal groups are not developed by management, although they are a fact of managerial life. Why do individuals form informal groups within the formal organizational structure? It is important to remember that informal groups cannot exist without a formal structure. As we discussed previously, individuals have a series of needs. Some of these needs can be met by the formal structure, some can be met through various activities that are beyond the work setting. However, some needs can be met by the informal groups in the working environment.

In a very basic sense, individuals have a need to affiliate with other individuals. The informal group provides a viable mechanism for this to occur. This need can often be simple, or it can be quite complex. In either case research by Mayo (1933) has shown that lack of opportunity for social contact has resulted in employees perceiving their jobs to be unsatisfying. In addition, the individual has needs of self-esteem that can be met partially through coworkers' and colleagues' recognition. Certainly feedback from management in a formal sense greatly assists in the development of self-image, but the informal feedback of others on the unit is a most gratifying experience. This kind of emotional underpinning produces a degree of stability for the individual and assists in the development of a positive attitude toward self and work. Likewise, constructive advice from fellow employees that assists in the execution of assigned responsibilities without the awareness of management is a moving force to concrete relationships among members on a unit. Thus, the individual has many needs that can be helped through identification with an informal group in the working environment.

MANAGEMENT OF INFORMAL GROUPS

The nurse-manager functions in an environment that is not just the formal organization but, rather, a complex combination of the formal and informal organization. This complex combination constitutes reality. In every organizational setting there are informal groups operating. However, the key question for nurse-managers is how philosophically these informal groups should be viewed. Should they be considered as deviates from the formal authority structure? Should they be considered as totally detrimental to the operation of the nursing unit? How can managers work to eradicate this clandestine aspect of management life?

Given the fact of the existence of the informal group, it can be stated that the action of the informal group is at variance with any activity authorized by formal management. Before we can make any value judgements about this deviation, we should examine the various aspects of informal groups. Do they bring any positive aspects to the overall management of the unit?

We know from previous discussions that the informal group is helpful to the individual in the areas of self-image, identification, affiliation, and increased emotional stability. Thus, it could be said that the informal group provides a base for social satisfaction. The individual then should have a more positive emotional foundation with, rather than without, the informal group. This situation should result in lower employee turnover and greater satisfaction with the job. Thus, this aspect of the informal group provides a positive moving force for management.

The informal group has its own communication network known as the grapevine. Some managers try to cut off communicaions through the grapevine because it is not the formal channel of communication. However, more astute managers identify the source of the grapevine and use this channel to enhance overall effectiveness of the unit. Davis, (1967, p. 224) has found that grapevines have been accurate conveyors of information 75 percent of the time if the information is noncontroversial organizational data. Many managers feel that the grapevine is not very accurate primarily due to the fact that the errors have a longer lasting impression. This unfavorable reputation of the grapevine comes from rumors which, by definition, are not based on fact. As rumors arise on the unit, they should be handled by the nurse-manager in a firm manner and on a consistent basis with sensitivity. The nurse-manager would make a strategic error by attacking the grapevine itself. The grapevine can be a valuable asset to management if used in a prudent and proper way.

One of the most crucial tests for management is to ascertain if the informal group is positively assisting management in the accomplishment of organizational goals and objectives. In many cases the informal group working as a team on the unit can greatly facilitiate the attainment of objectives through a combined work effort. On the unit, working at the bedside and interfacing with other ancillary systems, members of the informal group can identify and isolate areas in the formal structure that have either not been fully thought out or simply not anticipated. As a result, they can fill the gaps in the formal structure and assist in the overall effectiveness of the unit. Likewise, the more the informal group on the unit works as a team, the less supervision is needed, and the manager can experience an actual increase in the span of control. As a result of these positive factors, the informal group can produce a more effective environment and enhance the management of the unit.

Informal groups are a disadvantage if they operate to decrease the overall effectiveness of the unit: Work is not as productive as it should be, an increased amount of supervision is needed, and results expected are less predictable. Likewise, the amount of control exerted is greater than originally conceived under the formal structure.

If nurse-managers are to be effective in dealing with the informal group, they must develop a positive philosophy toward it and design a plan of action to deal with it. French (1963) conducted research about dealing with informal groups and concluded that, in fact, management can exercise influence over them.

In accordance with a positive philosophical approach, managers should work with the informal group and not against it. Every effort should be made to convey understanding and acceptance while attempting to integrate the group more into the formal structure. During the decision-making process, nurse-managers should consider the possible implications on the informal group. These implications can greatly assist in the final implementation of decisions because of the possible positive and supportive nature of the informal group. But in all cases, it must be remembered that the formal structure must prevail as the primary organizational vehicle, whereas the informal structure should act to support and enhance the organizational effort.

SUMMARY

Individuals have needs that must be satisfied in the organizational setting. We know that in making assignments on a nursing unit, there must be goodness of fit between the situation and the needs of the individual. Some of these needs of the individual are met through the working environment.

While working on the unit, the individual interacts with others to develop informal groups. Thus, these informal groups result from activities related to job performance that are not prescribed by the formal organization. Informal groups are not developed by management, although they are a fact of managerial life. They cannot exist without a formal structure preceding them chronologically. Informal groups are usually helpful to the individual's self-image, identification, affiliation, and increased emotional stability.

It is well recognized that the activities of informal groups are at variance with any activity authorized by formal management. The informal group develops its own communication network known as the grapevine, which is outside the formal communication channel designed by management.

Informal groups can be a positive factor on management operation by increasing work productivity, reducing supervision required, increasing the span of control needed, filling formal organization gaps, and resulting in better management. Likewise, the informal group can decrease overall effectiveness, increase supervision required, decrease span of control, and hinder accomplishment of organizational goals.

The astute nurse-manager should develop a positive attitude toward informal groups, work with and not against them, try to integrate the group more into the formal structure, and be supportive. In all cases the formal structure must prevail, and the informal should complement and assist that organizational effort.

BIBLIOGRAPHY

Argyris, Chris. *Integrating the Individual and the Organization*. New York: Wiley, 1964.

Berelson, Bernard, and Steiner, Gary A. *Human Behavior: An Inventory of Scientific Findings*. New York: Harcourt, Brace and World, 1964.

Davis, Keith. *Human Relations at Work,* 3rd ed. New York: McGraw-Hill, 1967.

Elbing, Alvar D. *Behavioral Decisions in Organizations*. Glenview, Ill.: Scott, Foresman, 1970.

French, Cecil L. "Some Structural Aspects of a Retail Sales Group." *Human Organization* (Summer 1963) 146–151.

Hampton, David R.; Sumner, Charles E.; and Webber, Ross A. *Organizational Behavior and the Practice of Management*. Glenview, Ill.: Scott, Foresman, 1968.

Homans, George C. *The Human Group*. New York: Harcourt, Brace and World, 1950.

Mayo, Elton. *The Human Problems of an Industrial Civilization*. Cambridge, Mass.: Harvard University Press, 1933.

Rogers, Carl R. *On Becoming a Person*. Boston: Houghton Mifflin, 1961.

Chapter 11

Sociopolitical Forces in Nursing

We have examined the informal aspects of organizations as they evolve. It is important for nurse managers to delve deeper into the reality of the operating environment to understand better the complexities of management and organizational life. There are certain social and political dimensions that enhance nurse-managers' effectiveness. These dimensions comprise a significant portion of the social systems of organizations. They obtain their being from both the formal and informal aspects of organization, with the individuals in the organization being primarily responsible for relationships that evolve through these dimensions.

STATUS SYSTEMS

One of the most important social dimensions in organizations is status. The status of an individual represents the social rank of a person in relation to others in the social system. Status can be subdivided into formal and informal status. Formal status is usually identified by the rank of individuals as provided by the authority structure of the organization. Informal status is the individual's social rank, which results from others' perceptions.

An individual seeking employment in a nursing unit will bring with him or her a certain degree of status from sources outside the organization itself. Thus, the characteristics of the individual can be considered as input factors of status. These characteristics include education, age, race, religion, sex, family, competence, and friends. From a societal point of view, generally more status is given to the more educated, the older, the more competent, and to males. These views are based in society and are in a continual state of flux. The role of women has been changing substantially since World War II and this has accelerated during the 1960s and early and mid-1970s. Likewise, status hierarchies exist among races, religions, and family origins.

In addition to individual characteristics, which should be considered, one also must recognize the relative prestige of the occupation and prestige of the service or product produced. In the case of service or product, Campbell (1960) reported that medical services received the highest ranking of prestige among college students surveyed in Ohio. Within the services delivered in health and medical care, where does nursing stand from a prestige standpoint? What constitutes its prestige level?

Lysaught (1970, p. 58) reports that three concepts of nursing practice exist. He states that "these three concepts include the lay public's generally global view of a nurse; the occupational view of the nurse held by physicians, administrators, and some nurses; and the view of an increasing number of nurses, and some other health personnel, who regard nursing as an emerging profession."

In summary, the lay view supports the social importance of nursing, the occupational stresses technical competencies and skill, whereas the professional emphasizes thinking and judgement. Thus, the role and related status varies considerably in terms of the referent group. Ideally all referent groups could become more aligned with the last group, but that requires much time, effort, education, and commitment. The current level of ambiguity was recently noted by Anderson (1968) when he observed that the role of the physician appears well defined but that the role of the nurse is ambiguous. This situation may have become more confused since that time with the designation of the clinical nurse specialist, nurse clinician, and nurse practitioner. As mentioned earlier, it certainly would seem that the role of the nurse is unclear; however, the direction of change is quite clear—toward an expanded role.

It would appear that nursing from a sociological point of view is becoming more instrumental in relation to expression. Actions that are directly related toward goals and objectives are considered instrumental, whereas those activities that assist in maintaining motivational equilibrium among individuals in the group are defined generally as expressive. This is the case in doctors' well-defined roles; perhaps the role interaction may clarify or perhaps further confuse the status of the two health-care provider groups. It would appear that as the expanded role becomes more prevalent that role and functions of the nurse become more instrumental. Thus, the relative status level of nursing should become higher because of the more direct action toward goal attainment in contrast to only maintaining motivational equilibrium among individuals in the group.

The organization is the primary source of formal status. The principal factor within the organizational structure that causes status is the organizational level. The level represents the official rank that an individual has in the formal structure. An individual of higher rank has more authority in a formal sense and, as a result of that rank, can make decisions affecting other individuals of lower rank.

In addition to organizational level, other factors must be considered. These status factors include seniority, type of work, conditions of work, and the compensation level. Certainly nurses who have been on the unit longer and who have worked in the hospital longer would be afforded higher status. It is reasoned that in general they know the "ropes," know how to get things done quicker working through others, and have established working relationships with physicians and the various ancillary departments within the hospital. The type of nursing care required is usually a differentiating factor in status determinations. The greater the skill required as well as the extent of the decision-making role of a nurse in caring for patients will be a positive force of elevating status. Foley (1975) provides a case in point. In his article entitled "Doctorette" (I am not sure I like the title), he describes a new superstar on the medical team. He states that "she is the intensive care nurse. She is young, intelligent, energetic, and talented, but she has to be. She works mentally and physically at full speed for eight hours. . . . Floor nurses think she is a snob" (p. 86). This article is a good example of how the type of work can be a differentiating factor in status. As can be seen, increased status does not always concomitantly provide popularity.

Generally, better working conditions also increase status. For example, the nurse-manager who is director of nursing usually has an office that is larger and more elaborately furnished than does the nurse-manager who is a unit director, and it is usually located in a place that is quieter and closer to the top administrators' offices. This increased level of status is also apparent in a school of nursing where the dean might have a larger corner office with windows, whereas an assistant professor may have room enough for a desk, chair, visitor chair, and a filing cabinet. So it is important to watch for these evidences of status in attempting to identify the status level of individuals in the organization.

An individual's compensation level depends on many factors and is a status symbol in itself. Usually the greater the skill level and decision-making authority, the greater the seniority, and the better the working conditions, the higher the compensation level. The way compensation levels are computed within a nursing department will provide evidence of increased status. The differing levels may include punching of a time clock, signing a time sheet, or not having to provide any evidence. Notice in this respect that moving up the organizational structure, the managerial approach to verifying working attendance goes from Theory X to Theory Y, in other words, from a situation of more control to less control.

Barnard (1948) has suggested that status developed in organizations does produce some stratifications of organizations. It also makes the structure less flexible. However, status can result in positive aspects for the individual and the organization. The status provided to the individual assists in meeting ego needs, and the organization can enhance its communication process. In addition, status can act as a motivating factor for nurse-managers. In some situations (for the hours worked), a nurse-manager may receive less compensation than an individual lower in the hierarchy, but the position and related responsibility and authority can be greatly offsetting factors in the determination of status and manager satisfaction.

AUTHORITY AND POWER SYSTEMS

McClelland and Burnham (1976, p.100) reported that "contrary to what one might think, a good manager is not one who needs personal success or who is people oriented, but one who likes power."

Power emanates from many sources both from inside and outside the organization. Authority is a part of power and issues from the formal organization. Authority then can be viewed as power from the organization as a result of position, organizational level, and responsibilities. This type of power is granted to the manager from an individual higher in the organizational setting. Power of this nature may be considered as formal power.

However, power as a concept is much wider in scope than just formal power. In addition to formal power, there exists informal power. This form of power can come from the personality of the manager, colleagues, perceived competency, and a willingness of individuals on the unit to perform. The fact that an individual nurse-manager is granted formal power by the organization does not ensure that individuals on the unit will respond. Power represents a relationship between individuals on the unit and among units. It is the manager's ability to influence others into action that constitutes power. In *Management and Machiavelli* Jay (1967) states that "real power does not lie in documents and memos outlining your terms of reference and area of jurisdiction: it lies in what you can achieve in practice."

In his famous work *The Functions of the Executive,* Barnard (1938, p.100) insightfully states that "the decision as to whether an order has authority or not lies with the persons to whom it is addressed and does not reside in 'persons of authority' or those who issue these orders . . ." The concept that Barnard is conveying is most important and must be understood for nurse-managers to be effective. It is the process of obtaining power whereby individuals in the organization delegate power *upward* to the manager. In other words, formal power as granted by management will essentially be without power unless it is accepted by those individuals working in the unit. This observation will become even more critical as nursing-care delivery continues to become more specialized and complex. Flippo (1970, p.727) addresses this type of problem but he states that "the formal right to manage . . . has remained, but the capacity to manage it has been diluted and spread among a number of experts. The man who knows has power regardless of the formal organization."

The nature of power is such that it does not have an upper limit of amount, and when used collectively it will be stronger than the sum of power of individuals acting independently. In many organizations the informal aspects of power can be seen by developing a sociogram of interactions within the organization. These diagrams can indicate where the sources of true power lie in the organization. It is interesting to compare a sociogram to a formal organization chart to see the effects that overall power has on the perceived formal power structure of the organization. These kinds of exercises are helpful to nursing management in stressing less formal power and in seeking cooperation from other power-source individuals in moving toward the attainment of organizational goals. Certainly, knowing the power structure will greatly keep nurse-managers from appearing too "green" and should help prevent strategic errors in carrying out responsibilities.

ORGANIZATIONAL POLITICAL SYSTEMS

Hampton, Sumner, and Webber (1968, p.588) have stated that "strategic behavior in organizations takes the form of 'playing politics,' propaganda activities, withholding information, the display of power (or the concealing of it) and other such actions."

Organizational political systems comprise what we observe as strategic behavior. It is through strategic behavior that nurse-managers are involved in the politics of the unit and the hospital. Pfiffner and Sherwood, (1960, p. 311) have described this political process environment as "the network of interaction by which power is acquired, transferred, and exercised upon others."

Nurse-managers must be astutely aware that power represents both formal and informal power. Consequently, they have formal power from the organization and power from other sources. However, the power total is comprised of their power and other power that is diffused throughout the organization. Therefore, when managers attempt to move on an issue, the power moves into action, and the end result will be politics. From a theoretical standpoint, if total insight into the effects of actions could be forecast with great accuracy, then the resultant politics should be of minor magnitude. In actual nursing practice, this is very seldom the case.

Thus, when power moves into action nurse-managers can anticipate conflict on the unit and/or with other departments. Conflict will result because when action has occurred through the use of power, some change is being introduced into the environment. Individuals and departments will react to the change depending on its extent and magnitude and their perceptions of its beneficial or detrimental aspects. Some reactions to change are negative because it is change, without evaluations of the possible benefits that may be derived from such change. Others will react to change negatively if their perception is that it will be detrimental to their own power and status. Certainly the extent of resultant conflict must be controlled, since excessive conflict can be quite damaging to the effective operation of the unit and/or department. This level of conflict can often do more harm than good to the organization. On the other hand, if the proposed change will enhance power and status of existing power sources, they will diligently work to effectuate the change. More on concepts of change will be covered in a later chapter.

How does the resolution of conflict occur over time? When the change is introduced, the individual, unit, and department are being requested to adjust to and to accommodate the change. The approach used by nurse-managers is most crucial to effectuate the change. As a minimum, nurse-managers should provide the rationale for the change and indicate how it will enhance the effectiveness of the organization. This is one of the most common complaints that I have heard about proposed changes: "No reason was given, we were just told to do it. If a reason was asked for, the response was that the director of nursing wants it done that way, or administration has issued an edict so we must comply." This approach of not providing appropriate rationale is one of the best ways to ensure conflict and resistance to the change.

If the change is properly conveyed, then adjustment will occur and accommodation can be achieved through a series of trade-offs. In some cases, this may entail the slight losing of controls, perhaps the incentive of rewards, or possibly a present or future exchange of favors. At all times nurse-managers must be calculating the trade-offs to ensure that the goal of change is secured without sacrificing too much or without grossly curtailing the management prerogatives of future issues.

In the operational environment nurse-managers are faced with many areas of politics. These can occur between managers. Such a situation is evidenced by the frequent struggle for nursing personnel either through a nursing office or the personnel office. When budgets are tight—as they are in most cases—conflict will arise over budget allocations between departments and units. Additional conflict can be seen in the case of promotions where heavy budgetary constraints permit limited promotion even though greater promotion potential exists.

Nurse-managers must also perform well politically in the arena of personnel reporting to the manager. As mentioned earlier, managers must secure the approval of power from organization members lower in the formal structure to ensure effective management. Unions have developed in the hospital setting in recent years. This represents a concerted effort by organizational members who are not in management to secure a greater voice in the operation of the organization. This area is a difficult one for nurse-managers. In many cases nurse-managers were among the non-management members of the organization before promotion. To assist nurse-managers in understanding these developments, a chapter is devoted to this topic later in this book.

Another area of responsibility is the relationship with nonnursing departments, such as pharmacy, x-ray, etc. In this case politics usually evolve through attempts by nursing to respond to physician orders and meet patients' needs on a timely basis. The politics involved in this arena primarily consist of attempting to obtain desired results while under stress and not appearing to exhibit that condition. This type of approach can be most beneficial and productive, but certainly requires an understanding of self prior to understanding others.

SUMMARY

To understand better the complexities of management and organizational life, nurse-managers must delve into the reality of the operating environment. The social and political dimensions of the organization must be examined. These dimensions can be viewed through the following systems: status, authority and power, and organizational political systems.

Status represents the social rank of an individual in relation to others in the social system. Status is derived from both formal and informal areas. Formal status emanates from the organization, whereas informal is secured from other sources.

Power is obtained from many sources both inside and outside the organization. Authority is power from the organization as a result of position, organizational level, and responsibilities. Other forms of power, usually referred to as informal power, come from the personality of the manager, colleagues, perceived competency of the manager, and a willingness of individuals on the unit to perform. The last aspect is important because individuals in the organization delegate power upward to the manager. Thus, power granted by management will essentially be without power unless it is accepted by those individuals working on the unit. Power does not have an upper limit, and when individuals act collectively their power is greater than that of each individual.

Organizational political systems comprise what we observe as strategic behavior. This behavior constitutes what is called politics. The political process is a network of interactions, which provide the delivery mechanism for power whether it is gained, given, or exercised upon others. When power moves into action, politics and conflict result. This conflict is usually resolved over time through adjustment and accommodation. Accommodation is generally accompanied by trade-offs. The nurse-manager operates in many areas of politics, including manager to manager, manager to managed, and manager to nonnursing departments.

BIBLIOGRAPHY

Anderson, O. W. *Toward an Unambiguous Profession? A Review of Nursing*. Chicago: Center for Health Administration Series, No. A6, 1968.

Barnard, Chester I. *The Functions of the Executive*. Cambridge, Mass.: Harvard University Press, 1938.

————. *Organization and Management*. Cambridge, Mass.: Harvard University Press, 1948.

Campbell, Robert E. "The Prestige of Industries." *Journal of Applied Psychology* (February 1960): 1–5.

Flippo, Edwin B. *Management: A Behavioral Approach*, 2nd ed. Boston: Allyn & Bacon, 1970.

Foley, Thomas J. "Doctorette." *Journal of Surgery, Gynecology and Obstetrics* 141 (July 1975): 86.

Hampton, David R.; Sumner, Charles E.; and Webber, Ross A. *Organizational Behavior and the Practice of Management*. Glenview, Ill.: Scott, Foresman, 1968.

Jay, Antony. *Management and Machiavelli*. New York: Holt, Rinehart and Winston, 1967.

Lysaught, Jerome P. *An Abstract for Action*. New York: McGraw-Hill, 1970.

McClelland, David C., and Burnham, David H. "Power Is the Great Motivator." *Harvard Business Review*, vol. 54, no. 2 (March–April 1976): 100–110.

Pfiffner, John M., and Sherwood, Frank P. *Administrative Organization*. Englewood Cliffs, N.J.: Prentice-Hall, 1960.

Chapter 12

Effects of Specialization
in Nursing

We have examined some informal aspects of organizations and sociopolitical forces in nursing. Now, as a final aspect of the behavioral influences on organizing in nursing, we shall consider the effects of specialization in nursing.

The specialization that we observe in nursing has evolved through technological advances in medicine and the proliferation of specialties in the practice of medicine. Certainly, the technological advances have resulted in a great diversification of medical sources and personnel. Stevens (1971, p. 2) recently stated that "the full potential of medicine cannot be transmitted to an individual without a panoply of facilities bristly with equipment, and an army of specialized health personnel; and this is increasingly true of routine medical diagnosis as well as esoteric treatment."

The role of the physician has thus become more and more dependent on allied health personnel as the advances in technology have made the specialization in the practice of medicine a more pronounced fact of health-care delivery. Wilson (1959–60, p. 178) observed this phenomenon when he stated, "what is important is the analysis of a trend in the organizational structure of the hospital which has affected and is affecting the scope and texture of the doctor's role therein. His role as unchallenged master, what might be considered as a charismatic role, is changing. The seemingly irreversible process of specialization means that one vital quality of charismatic roles, their global vigor and assumed diffuse efficacy, is severely foreshortened." Thus, increasing medical specialization has curtailed the autonomy of the physician.

The reduction of autonomy has increased the dependency of the physician on nursing and other health professionals. Consequently, the physician acting as a member of the team finds his performance heavily dependent on the effective interactions and competencies of the other members of the team, particularly nurses. Thus, it was a natural evolution that the role and function of the nurse would be expanded and professionalized. This process of specialization in nursing has produced certain stresses and strains within the profession itself. Issues that face nursing as a result of specialization include the delineation of specialists, the type and length of education needed, the licensing and certification specialization requires, and how the different ranks will professionally interrelate. Considerable effort is currently being devoted to these key questions by professional associations, boards of nursing, and state and federal legislatures.

FUNCTIONAL DIFFERENTIATION

Previously we considered the concepts of job design, which indicated that similar functions can be grouped in establishing position descriptions. This condition continues to be true, but as a result of functional differentiation (specialization), many more separate and distinct functions exist. For nurse-managers, specialization of function and staff has greatly increased the complexity of their role. Donabedian (1973, p. 280) states that "the effect of functional differentiation [specialization] on interchangeability and substitutability is interestingly complicated." The problem increases as nurse-managers move up the authority structure of the hospital. The direct management concern in this area is the staffing problem and the assignment of nursing personnel. Prior to the proliferation of specialists, nurses could be assigned to different parts of the hospital without an overriding concern for differences in nursing care required. However, with increased specialization, a nurse-manager would most likely be doing a disservice to the nurse and the patient, by assigning a nurse who has always worked on a medical floor to a neonatal intensive-care unit. The ability to assign nursing personnel at random to patients has been greatly precluded due to the functional differentiation that has occurred. Certainly, some possibilities of interchangeability and substitution exist, but the extent of such activity in general has been voluntarily curtailed by prudent nurse-managers.

Up to this point, we have been considering nurses who have gained knowledge through specialized continuing education courses and experience. Now we will discuss the role of the clinical nurse specialist with preparation at the master's degree level.

CLINICAL NURSE SPECIALIST

In considering the role of the clinical nurse specialist, the nurse-manager's job is more complex. Nurse-managers must understand the role and capability of clinical nurse specialists. The education of the specialist is at the master's level. It would be nice at this point to give you a clear definition of the clinical nurse specialist, but this is not simple. Hummel (1972) reports that after reviewing 181 articles on clinical nurse specialists, the role is not clear. Hummel's work indicates that there is some consensus. Clinical nurse specialists would be involved in direct patient care, interdisciplinary activities, developing innovative and experimental approaches to patient care, consultation, and staff development. All activities identified were specified by 80 percent or more of the articles except for staff development, which occurred in 66 percent of the cases. Thus, the general areas of the role are identified.

Brown (1971, p. 69) has perhaps one of the best definitions for the clinical nurse specialist and provides some insights from an organizational point of view regarding this role. The clinical nurse specialist is "generally outside the organizational line on the chart in order to move where and when she thinks she is most needed. She is a consultant who acts as a practitioner, teacher, and supervisor; her primary role in cooperation with the physician may be viewed as that of representative of the patient's interest within the concept of comprehensive coordinated and continuing care."

Dirschel (1976, p. 1–11) reports that the clinical nurse specialist has primary functions, which include role model, collaborator with members of an interdisciplinary team, change agent, teacher (staff and patient), and consultant.

Nurse-managers must realize that in many cases the clinical nurse specialist, in acting as a consultant, works for the director of nursing and acts as staff support to the unit. The specialist has power from knowledge and can be a most valuable asset to the unit. We know that in terms of quality of care (Donabedian, 1969, p. 221) that specialists are more likely to deliver care of higher quality than do generalists. This appears true for physicians through "medical care appraisal." It is also apparently true for the clinical nurse specialist. Studies conducted by Simms (1965), Little

(1967), Georgopolous and Christman (1970), and Barrett (1972) support the concept of improvements in patient care as a result of the introduction of clinical nurse specialists to the patient care environment. Thus, nurse-managers should look to the specialist as the key staff resource to assist in the improvement of patient care.

NURSE MANAGER AND SPECIALIZATION

With the advent of specialization nurse-managers are faced with many challenges. They must realize that in general the specialist has more in-depth knowledge of the specialty than they do. But managers must know more about the overall situation including the specialty and other areas that interface with the specialty. The challenge of this managerial art increases as one rises in the formal organization structure.

As the dependency of the physician has increased relative to nursing, so has the dependency of the nurse manager who works with specialists in nursing. With increased dependency on staff, nurse-managers must be aware of the power and influence of the specialist as a result of acquired specialized knowledge. The situation makes it imperative that the specialist work *with* rather than strictly *for* the nurse manager. Certainly, nurse-managers retain final authority, but the authority role should not be used in a coercive manner with specialists. In general, managers should assume that specialists are self-motivated; therefore, managers should use Theory Y.

It is important for the nurse-manager to perceive a further under-standing of the specialist. As the specialist increases in knowledge in a specific area, the depth of knowledge in that area will obviously increase. However, with the increased depth of knowledge comes a form of func-tional fixation that precludes the viewing of the larger picture. In general, functional fixation in human behavior refers to the situation in which an individual attaches a meaning to an object and consequently is unable to see alternative meanings or applications (Duncker, 1945). Likewise, the areas of interest of the specialist appear to be reduced. Kornhauser (1962, p. 1) has suggested that specialist groups tend to foster a narrowing of perspectives, interests, and orientation, which tends to retard the ability of the members of a group to cooperate in an effective manner with other specialist groups. As a result of the limiting effect on breadth of knowl-edge versus depth of knowledge, the specialist tends to develop a certain ignorance with regard to other matters. Thus, the nurse-manager must remember the differences in perspectives between the manager and the specialist to deal effectively with this situation.

With the increased knowledge of the specialist comes a body of ter-minology that is sometimes unfamiliar to nurse-managers. As a result, a series of communication problems develops because the receiver (manager) does not have the same understanding of terminology as the sender (specialist). In many cases, nurse specialists can be quite impatient with managers over the lack of understanding. Specialists often demonstrate frustration if managers ask for the definitions of some terms. These communication problems must be overcome by nurse-managers through a persuasive approach of assisting specialists in the accomplishment of patient-care objectives.

In addition to communications problems, nurse-managers should consider the possible impact of specialization on fragmentation of care. With the proliferation of specialists, it is not uncommon to have a specialist who has in-depth knowledge of one body system. Consequently, the specialist often develops an orientation that precludes the identification of problems with other body systems. This situation results in the often-heard statement that no one is responsible for the whole patient. Wilson (1959–1960, p. 174) speaks philosophically to this type of situation, "The wise man appears not so wise when his knowledge shrinks—even if it coincidentally deepens—to some limited sphere; perhaps more precisely, his wisdom comes to resemble more a technical attribute, less an innate property of his person." To prevent this condition from developing, it is imperative that overspecialization to the possible detriment of the patient be prevented. Nurse-managers can alleviate this type of situation by permitting specialists of various areas to work together. In addition, providing an environment that will permit exchange of ideas and observations can help greatly in overcoming this problem. As might be expected a certain amount of cross-training through rotation of staff may be necessary. It is imperative that responsibility for the whole patient be assigned to the specialist with concomitant accountability for the quality of nursing care rendered to that patient.

INTEGRATION OF SPECIALISTS

The importance of nurse-managers' roles in the integration of specialists into the milieu of patient care cannot be overemphasized. Regardless of the specialist's knowledge, if the manager does not effectively assist in the integration process of the specialist, the impact of that specialized knowledge on patient care will not become a reality.

Simms (1965) and Schaefer (1973) have found that the impact of the nurse specialist on quality nursing care is heavily dependent on the nature and condition of employment. The greater the extent of nurse-manager support, the more likely that the system will provide mechanisms for specialist satisfaction and will enhance the quality of nursing care.

In other studies Scully (1967) and Smith (1971) report that nursing staff has shown considerable resistance to the integration of the nurse specialist in the unit. Problems from existing staff come from the perceived role of the specialist in the development of nursing-care plans (which is only an academic exercise performed by the students). Likewise, the problem of the divergent goals between the specialist and staff was an area of conflict. This related to the specialist's responsibility for staff development to establish similar goals for patient care.

Conflict between nurse-managers and specialists has been a barrier to integration of the specialist. Fagin (1967) and Edwards (1971) have provided observations with regard to this problem. Edwards reports that the head nurse feels threatened by the specialist. As a result, Fagin and Edwards suggest that perhaps the best solution to overcoming this threat and to effectuate the changes needed in nursing care is to have the specialist accept the authority position of the manager. The integration can be accomplished in this manner, but is the use of a specialist in a managerial position the best use of the specialized knowledge to enhance the quality of patient care? This approach certainly has definite advantages for the implementation of change, but there are also significant negative trade-offs with regard to the possible effective use of a specialist in direct patient care. Hopefully, time and experience will demonstrate the direction of this issue.

SUMMARY

This chapter considered the effects of specialization in nursing. The specialization that we observe in nursing has evolved through technological advances in medicine and the proliferation of specialties in the practice of medicine. This situation has resulted in the reduction of autonomy for the physician and an expanded role for nursing. The changing role of nurses is seen in the expanded roles, which manifested itself through continuing education and experience and through formal master's degree programs in nursing that permit an individual to attain the knowledge and status of the clinical nurse specialist.

Specialization of function and staff has greatly increased the complexity of the managers' roles. To a large extent, specialization has had a retardant effect on interchangeability and substitutability of staff.

The clinical nurse specialist presents an interesting opportunity and problem for the nurse-manager. The opportunity is the chance to improve the quality of nursing care on the unit through the efforts of this well-educated specialist. On the other hand, the clinical nurse specialist is generally outside the authority structure of the unit and in many cases may work directly for the director of nursing. In essence, the clinical nurse specialist is a staff resource to the manager and the unit staff, but this individual is not within that authority structure. Researchers have demonstrated that introducing the specialist to the patient-care environment does support the concept of improvements in patient care.

Other researchers report problems of communication and integration of the specialist. Studies have indicated that conflicts between nurse-managers and specialists have been a barrier to specialist integration. Suggestions were made that such integration could be effectuated by having the clinical nurse specialist perform the role of nurse-manager. It is apparent that regardless of the specialized knowledge received by the specialist, if the manager does not effectively assist in the integration process of the specialist, the impact of that specialized knowledge in patient care will not become a reality.

BIBLIOGRAPHY

Barrett, Jean. "The Nurse Specialist Practitioner: A Study." *Nursing Outlook* vol. 20, no. 8 (1972): 524–527.

Brown, Esther Lucile. *Nursing Reconsidered: A Study of Change*. Philadelphia: J. B. Lippincott, 1971.

Dirschel, Kathleen M. "The Conception, Gestation and Delivery of the Clinical Nursing Specialist." In *Quality Patient Care and the Role of the Clinical Nursing Specialist,* edited by Rachel Rotkovitch. New York: Wiley, 1976.

Donabedian, Avedis. *Aspects of Medical Care Administration: Specifying Requirements for Health Care*. Cambridge, Mass.: Harvard University Press, 1973.

————. *A Guide to Medical Care Administration, Vol II: Medical Care Appraisal—Quality and Utilization*. New York: American Public Health Association, 1969.

Duncker, Karl. "On Problem Solving." *Psychological Monographs,* vol. 58, no. 5 (1945).

Edwards, Jane. "Clinical Specialists Are Not Effective—Why?" *Supervisor Nurse* (August 1971): 39–47.

Fagin, Claire M. "The Clinical Specialist as Supervisor." *Nursing Outlook* (January 1967): 34–36.

Georgopolous, Basil, and Christman, Luther. "The Clinical Nurse Specialist: A Role Model." *American Journal of Nursing* (May 1970): 1030–1039.

Hummel, Patricia. "Identification of Different Approaches to Clinical Specialization in Graduate Education in Nursing." USPHS Division of Nursing Project, #1-D10-NU-09535-01, 1972.

Kornhauser, W. *Scientists in Industry: Conflict and Accommodation*. Berkeley: University of California Press, 1962.

Little, D. "The Nurse Specialists." *American Journal of Nursing* 67 (1967): 552.

Schaefer, Jeanne A. "The Satisfied Clinician: Administrative Support Makes the Difference." *Journal of Nursing Administration* (July–August 1973): 17–20.

Scully, Nancy Rae. "The Clinical Nursing Specialist: Practicing Nurse." *Nursing Outlook* (August 1965): 28–30.

Simms, L. L. "The Clinical Nurse Specialist: An Experiment." *Nursing Outlook,* vol. 13, no. 8 (August 1965): 26–28.

Smith, Margaret L. "The Clinical Specialist: Her Role in Staff Development." *Journal of Nursing Administration* (January–February 1971): 33–36.

Stevens, Rosemary. *American Medicine and the Public Interest.* New Haven: Yale University Press, 1971.

Wilson, Robert N. "The Physician's Changing Hospital Role." *Human Organization,* vol. 18, no. 4 (Winter 1959–1960): 177–183.

Directing in Nursing

Part Four discusses concepts relating to the formal directing function in nursing, including nursing leadership, effective performance appraisal systems, and continuing education in nursing (Section A). The behavioral influences on this directing function are reviewed through the involvement process in nursing, communication process in nursing, and effective group dynamics in nursing.

Chapter 13 covers the characteristics of leadership in managers, followership, and the integration of leadership and followership. In addition, leadership styles are examined to include motivational and power styles. The primary power styles examined are autocratic, laissez faire, and participative styles. In addition, the specific managerial problems of the front-line nurse-manager are reviewed.

Chapter 14 examines an effective performance appraisal system for nursing. Topics covered include performance appraisal considerations, rewards systems, and the appraisal process. The process as discussed is based on a system of management by objectives.

Chapter 15 considers the need for continuing education of nurse managers and staff. Areas of concern are inservice education, external education, nature of nurse-manager development, approaches to nurse-manager development, philosophy of continuing education, and the evaluation of continuing education.

Chapter 16 considers the involvement process in nursing. Concepts necessary for an effective involvement process include a motivational base, influence, involvement inputs on positions, and involvement and the organizational environment.

Chapter 17 examines the communication process in nursing. Topics included on this important subject are components of communication and effectiveness, responsibility and accountability, formal and informal information systems, message considerations, preparedness and evaluation, and general communication considerations. The final areas of concern are the nurse-manager and the grapevine and communication and emotion.

The final chapter on the directing functions examines group dynamics in nursing. Discussion areas are advantages of groups, disadvantages of groups, considerations for effective groups, and nursing conferences. The nursing conferences considered are beginning of shift conferences, case conferences, report conferences, and the problem-solving conference.

Formal Directing

Chapter 13

Formal Nursing Leadership

We have considered the first two functions of management—namely planning and organizing. Now we will examine the third function of directing. The formal aspects are to be covered first, followed by the informal aspects. In the formal portion, the concepts of formal nursing leadership, reward systems in nursing, and management education in nursing will be considered. Now we shall examine the concept of formal nursing leadership.

As mentioned in Chapter 1, management consists of planning, organizing, directing, and controlling. Leadership is one part of directing that also encompasses rewards systems, management education, involvement, and communication processes, as well as effective group dynamics. The fact that leadership is a part of directing does not imply that leadership is not important. On the contrary, leadership is an essential ingredient to effective directing and managing. Excellent planning can often occur with the development of a well-conceived organizing process, but if the appropriate leadership cannot be brought to bear on the operations of the organization and unit, much of the anticipated effectiveness cannot be realized. Without effective leadership, the organization and the unit will be just a collection of health personnel, patients, and equipment. Nursing leadership is the ability of the nurse-manager to convince other unit personnel to work toward the attainment of the organization, unit, and patient-care objectives. Nurse-managers constitute the sole unifying force to bring individuals on a unit together to work effectively within the organizational structure. It is only through leadership that individuals will be drawn together and be motivated toward the attainment of goals. Leadership, then, is the unifying and motivating force that brings reality to the unit from a stage of mere potential.

A review of the literature indicates that many articles and books have been written about leadership (Tead, 1935; Selznick, 1957; Tannenbaum & Schmidt, 1958; Bennis, 1959; Schlotfeld, 1963; Mann, 1964; Korn, 1966; McGregor, 1966; Miller, 1971; Fry & Lauer, 1972; Alexander, 1972; Douglass & Bevis, 1974). Even though much information is available on leadership, very little is known about what makes an effective leader. Personal traits have been studied for some time as an indicator of the effective manager; studies have been conducted about the role behavior of the manager; and a considerable amount of information was published regarding the various managerial styles that can be used. Many articles have also been written about the supervisor in nursing with an entire journal being devoted to this aspect of nursing (i.e., *Supervisor Nurse*).

We shall now consider various aspects of leadership in nursing.

CHARACTERISTICS OF LEADERSHIP IN MANAGERS

Research has been conducted to establish the characteristics that make an effective leader. The early work addressed the manager; later work examined the individuals who work for the manager. Subsequently, research has been directed toward the complexity of the environment encompassing leader, followers, and situations.

Predictive models were based on such aspects of the manager as graphology, phrenology, and astrology (Davis, 1967). These approaches came into vogue and did not produce the long-range predictability as originally conceived.

A series of research efforts was devoted to demographic studies with the hope that background, education, and other factors would yield a model useful for effective prediction of potential managers through the selection process. Over 60 years of research did not provide significant insight into the prediction of manager success (Taylor, 1960).

Many managers are perceived as natural leaders because they exhibit charismatic leadership qualities. Florence Nightingale's leadership characteristics were described as follows (*Eminent Victorians,* 1948, p. 148):

> As for her voice, it was true of it, even more than of her countenance, that it had that in it "one must fain call master." Those clear tones were in no need of emphasis: "I never heard her raise her voice," said one of her companions. "Only, when she had spoken, it seemed as if nothing could follow but obedience.' Once, when she had given some direction, a doctor ventured to remark that the thing could not be done. "But it must be done," said Miss Nightingale. A chance bystander, who heard the words, never forgot through all his life the irresistible authority of them. And they were spoken quietly—very quietly indeed.

Through situations such as that described above, research was conducted to find the characteristics (traits) that make a successful manager. As more and more research was performed to establish such traits, the listing became larger and larger. The results of the studies produced a general lack of consensus among those conducting the research and minimal correlational relationships (Bennis, 1959).

Some characteristics of successful managers have been described in studies. These may be summarized as follows: intelligence, social maturity and breadth, inner motivation, and human relations attitude (Davis, 1967, p. 99).

These characteristics indicate that the manager who has a greater understanding of people is more successful. Those managers who are more emotionally stable and demonstrate maturity have greater self-assurance and command respect. Likewise, those of higher intellectual ability tend to be good managers. Managers who possess a higher drive toward goal attainment and accomplishment have greater motivation and are more successful. These characteristics appear to be more true of managers higher in the organizational structure than lower in the structure.

FOLLOWERSHIP

It seems apparent that the personal characteristics of a leader vary and depend on many other factors. Thus, as McGregor (1966, p. 73) so aptly states, "leadership is not a property of the individual, but a complex relationship among . . . variables." The obvious question must be raised: Can you be a leader without any followers? From an authority point of view, Barnard (1938) states that "the decision as to whether an order has authority or not lies with the persons to whom it is addressed, and does not reside in 'persons of authority' or those who issue these orders." It is most important that this concept be understood by nurse-managers. For without such acceptance by others, leaders have no followers and essentially are powerless.

Koontz and O'Donnell (1974, p. 355) indicate a similar orientation toward leadership when they state as an integral part of the principle of leadership that "since people tend to follow those in whom they see a means of satisfying their own personal goals, the more a manager understands what motivates his subordinates and how these motivations operate, and the more he reflects these in carrying out his managerial actions, the more effective as a leader he is likely to be." Thus, the imperative charge for a nurse-manager to become a leader is in providing the necessary mechanisms for motivation of individuals on the unit or in the department such that they will follow the lead that you provide for them.

INTEGRATION OF LEADERSHIP AND FOLLOWERSHIP

As more and more research evidence became general knowledge, it was apparent that characteristics of leaders did not provide much needed answers to organizational success. The exclusive focus on what mechanisms motivate employees also seems to demonstrate a high degree of variability from one department to another and from one unit to another (Herzberg, 1975, pp. 361–376). Thus, the simplistic view of only the leader or only the employee was insufficient to provide the degree of predictability originally hoped for by the management researchers. As is often true in life, the answer must lie in a complex approach to the problem. Specifically what we observe are the leader and followers interacting in a series of situations that collectively comprise the environment.

We know that the leader and followers must find sources of satisfaction from their working environment. The need structure of individuals was covered in detail earlier through the work primarily of Maslow (1954). Rice (1963) has concluded that organizations that provide conducive environments for employees, assist those employees greatly in dealing realistically and effectively with their jobs and thereby provide sources of psychological and social satisfaction. Managers who operate in a favorable environment can also fulfill motives that they brought to the organizational setting. These motives are expressed as needs for achievement, affiliation, and power (McClelland, 1961; McClelland & Burnham, 1976).

In an attempt to examine the environmental aspects of the situation, Korman (1966) reports two dimensions that the leader must consider to provide an appropriate setting for effectiveness. These dimensions have been defined as initiating structure and consideration. Basically, initiating structure refers to the degree to which management has structured the organization, including roles, tasks, and functions. Consideration primarily reflects the extent to which management has attempted to develop good interpersonal relationships with employees. It would appear that the greater the initiation of structure and the less consideration provided, the more employees would be precluded from satisfaction of needs; thus, the resulting motivational base would be minimal. Korman summarizes many studies that examined these concepts and concludes that little correlation exists as related to effectiveness.

Leadership involves a complex relationship among variables. In researching this problem Morse and Lorsch (1975, p. 379) conclude that management needs to move beyond Theory Y (McGregor, 1960). Their approach considered formal characteristics (i.e., the kind of task and the formal practice of the organization) and climate factors (i.e., perceptions and orientations of individuals to the organization). The climate characteristics included perception of structure, distribution of influence, relations with others, time orientation, and managerial style. Morse and Lorsch conclude that "managers can help this process by becoming more aware of what psychological needs seem to best fit the tasks available and the organizational setting, and by trying to shape personnel selection criteria to take account of these needs" (p. 388).

LEADERSHIP STYLES

Even though we recognize that the integration of leadership and followership into the organizational milieu is essential to effectiveness, it is also most helpful to examine some models of the practice of leadership that occur on the unit and in the department of nursing itself. These models will be expressed in terms of motivational styles and power styles.

MOTIVATIONAL STYLES

The way a nurse-manager approaches individuals on the unit will greatly determine the extent of motivation that will be exhibited by those individuals.

The two motivational styles are defined as positive and negative. Nurse-managers who use the positive motivational style will emphasize positive reinforcement mechanisms. These mechanisms can be expressed in many ways. The general attitudinal orientation provides a system of positive rewards. These rewards can range from a comment expressing pleasure with the excellent nursing care provided to the patient in Room 403 to a recommendation of a pay increase or promotion for an employee on the unit. It is important to provide feedback to individuals in the short-run as well as the long-run. Personnel on the unit need this positive feedback. In many cases, nurse-managers are under considerable pressure to direct resources effectively in a short timeframe and many times state that they only have time to intervene and correct problem areas. As a nurse-manager, you should take time—it doesn't really take that long—to thank a colleague for his or her work that day. Many nurse-managers are very surprised to learn that one of their best people has resigned—and they cannot understand why. In many cases, the individuals doing the best jobs on the unit are the ones most neglected; they do not need attention because they were not having problems. Beware of this common pitfall.

The second motivational style is the one used by nurse-managers who have a negative orientation toward individuals. This type of negative leadership can produce acceptable performance in many situations. But managers should be aware of the negative side effects that can be produced by this motivational style of leadership. The nurse-manager using this approach tends to stress penalties for not doing a good job. These penalties can be an oral reprimand in front of others on the unit. The nurse manager states directives with a threat or fear orientation up to and including dismissal. Thus, the nurse-manager will attempt to frighten individuals into doing a better job. With this approach, the individuals on the unit will spend a considerable amount of time attempting to protect themselves from the nurse-manager. In doing so, they will spend needless effort to cover their behavior and to document that whatever occurred must be someone else's fault. This behavior is to preclude a fear of reprimand or loss of face and to provide an element of job security.

It should be realized that nurse-managers use both positive and negative motivational styles of leadership. But overall a consistent model of being more positive or more negative usually surfaces over time. The more predominant motivational style will establish the overall attitude of individuals on the unit in terms of general expectations of their nurse-manager.

POWER STYLES

Previously we examined some sources of individual power. We noted that power came from multiple sources, which were categorized as formal and informal. We observed that through its organizing process the organization conveyed a formal power of position and this represented authority. The individual nurse working in a position of formal power brings to the position a certain amount of informal power as well. It is the collective power—informal and formal—that represents the total power that the nurse brings to the unit. At this point it is essential that we look at the various models of how power can be exercised in the unit and the department.

The manager's methods of influence (or use of power) can be categorized as follows: autocratic, laissez faire, and participative (or democratic). The original work to categorize these power styles of leadership was done by Lewin, Lippitt, and White.

The autocratic or authoritarian style is one in which the nurse-manager makes all decisions without seeking much input from individuals on the unit. This power style has been used in nursing for many years. It reflects a very directive type of leadership that stresses the giving of orders by the nurse-manager and the taking of orders by the other members of the unit. In this role the nurse-manager puts a high degree of emphasis on adherence to hospital policy and rules. Individuals are expected to follow orders as given, not to ask questions or to question authority, and the organizational system assumes the predominant role. As a result of this role behavior by the nurse-manager, individuals on the unit exhibit frustration primarily because mechanisms for satisfaction of individuals' needs have been thwarted by management. In many units the frustration level results from strict adherence to directives of the leadership, and apathy prevails because the individuals have not been properly integrated into the organizational environment. With increased apathy are the concomitant problems of motivation, morale, and certainly implications for the patient care.

The laissez faire style of leadership is at the opposite end of the continuum from the autocratic or authoritarian style. Under the laissez fair model, nurse-managers attempt to pass the role of decision making to the remaining members of the unit. In this role leaders do not accept the responsibility for decision making by asking the group to accept them as a member and for the group to make the decision. From a management standpoint, the leadership has been abdicated to the group with a resultant loss of direction and control. A great amount of freedom prevails for everyone because little formal structure exists. This leadership power style does not work well in nursing or any other discipline for that matter. In nursing, regardless of the level of staff ability and capability, the staff feels the need for some form of formal organizational structure. The directionless leadership of the group process in these cases tends to be long and tiring, without significant accomplishment, which does not necessarily enhance the need of staff for some degree of ego satisfaction.

The third model of power style is the participative or democratic approach. This model falls between the autocratic and laissez faire approaches. Nurse-managers attempt to seek extensive input from the members of the unit and thereby to a certain extent share with those members some of the responsibility for decision making. This style may be thought of as a consultative type of arrangement. Nurse-managers do not and cannot use this method for all decisions on the unit but, when possible, consult with unit members. Nurse-managers in this role usually develop group cohesiveness and commitment toward the accomplishment of goals by the members of the unit as they are further integrated into the organizational structure. This style permits individuals to express their views on problems, and through this participation process, they tend to identify more with the unit. From a leadership standpoint, it permits an exposure to more ideas, and allows more innovation than the autocratic approach, but nurse-managers must be careful to retain control. If control of the leadership role is not maintained by the nurse-manager, the management of the unit is likely to drift into a laissez faire situation. If utilized properly, the participative approach probably has the greatest potential for effectiveness. However, it is difficult to use because of the balance of power that occurs. In many units it can be described as tenuous at best.

In nursing management practice some variations of the three styles has been observed. The two most common variations are considered to be between the autocratic and participative styles. These variations have been labeled the benevolent autocratic and the manipulative autocratic. The benevolent autocratic desires to use the participative style but actually practices the autocratic style. In such cases nurse-managers attempt to secure acceptance of their decisions without really considering the input. The individuals on such units believe their leaders to be autocratic, whereas the leaders believe themselves to be democratic.

The manipulative autocratic attempts to make individuals perceive that they are truly participating in the decision-making process when in fact the decisions are being made by the leader. In this case, discussions are directed by the leader to reach the predetermined decision alternative.

In most nursing management situations a combination of leadership styles are exhibited. At the present time it appears that most nursing leaders are either benevolent autocrats or autocratic with some degree of participation.

FRONT-LINE NURSE MANAGER

Thus far we have discussed the role of the nurse-manager from a general management point of view. But it is now necessary that we make a distinction in levels of management. We know that supervision occurs at all levels of management in nursing. However, the role of the head nurse as manager is somewhat different from the other levels of management. Most of the other management positions in nursing are such that managers are supervising other managers. But head nurses are the only members of the management group who supervise nonmanagement personnel.

As a result, head nurses as nurse-managers must interact with two different groups. In an authority-reporting sense they work with managers. In a delegation-of-authority role they deal with subordinate personnel on the unit.

This role used to be considered a difficult one at best, but within the past few years the difficulty has become more exacerbated. The primary source of this increased difficulty has been the increase of union activity in nursing. Now more than ever front-line nurse-managers are placed in a position that has not been experienced before in the history of nursing management. Head nurses have always viewed their role as nurse and supervisor of other unit personnel. They belong to a national association that represents the profession, namely the ANA. Now, as a result of increased union activity, the job is being examined in greater detail. Do head nurses supervise others? Are they responsible for the evaluation of performance of others? Do they hire and fire personnel? If the majority of the responses are yes, then head nurses are members of management and cannot belong to any organization that may be involved in union activities at that hospital. This aspect and role of nurse-managers will be covered in greater detail later.

Front-line nurse-managers must perform the interesting and sometimes frustrating role of being the one in the middle. On the one hand, directives are being received from the nursing office and from administration to achieve certain goals of the organization. On the other hand, front-line nurse-managers receive pressure from the unit personnel in terms of individual needs, such as security, professional recognition, and professional independence as well as some opportunity to reduce paperwork and allow more time to care for patients. Nurse-managers know that their evaluation of a job well done will come from management. At the same time, if sufficient effort is not expended for the members of the unit, they may become somewhat uncooperative and frustrated and generally demonstrate a lack of acceptance and support of their manager.

In examining the role of first-line managers, Likert (1961) has researched their attitudes and productivity. He determined that managers could be divided into two categories—employee-centered and job-centered. The former group devoted primary attention to their employees, whereas the latter group were mostly interested in responding to their management. This research from industry indicates that employee-centered managers have better employee productivity and attitudes than do job-centered managers. Perhaps similar research in nursing might produce similar results. In any case, it is apparent that the role of the front-line supervisor is a difficult one indeed, and is become more difficult. As unions intervene more and more into the nursing milieu, the problems will only become greater and the job more difficult.

SUMMARY

Nursing leadership is the ability of nurse-managers to convince other unit personnel to work toward the attainment of the organization, unit, and patient care objectives. It is only through leadership that individuals will be drawn together to work effectively with the organizational structure.

Extensive research has been conducted to establish the characteristics (traits) of successful managers. Some of the more frequent characteristics are intelligence, social maturity and breadth, inner motivation, and human relations attitude. However, the results of studies produced a general lack of consensus among those conducting the research and minimal correlational relationships.

We noted that to be effective, leaders must have followers. For nurse-managers to become leaders, they must provide mechanisms for motivation of individuals on the unit in such a way that they will follow the lead that is provided for them.

Research concerning the leader only and the followers only was insufficient to provide the degree of predictability originally hoped for by the management researchers. The answer must lie in a complex approach to the problem, which includes the interactions of leaders and followers in a series of situations. Morse's and Lorsch's contingency theory appears most likely to suit this situation. This approach examines the fit between job, organization, and people.

We designated leadership styles as motivation styles and power styles. Motivational styles are either positive or negative representing the basic orientation of a leader toward employees. We defined power styles as autocratic, laissez faire and participative. In the autocratic style nurse-managers make all decisions without seeking much input from individuals on the unit. In the laissez faire approach, managers attempt to pass the role of decision making to the group. The third style is the participative model in which nurse-managers actively seek input from members of the unit and thereby to a certain extent share with those members some of the responsibility for decision making. Two variations of the three styles have been observed. These variations fall between autocratic and participative models and are called benevolent autocratic and manipulative autocratic. Most management situations exhibit a combination of leadership styles.

We reviewed the role of front-line nurse-managers and noted that they must interact with two different groups—managers and subordinates on the unit. The incursion of labor-union activity into the nursing milieu has exacerbated the difficulty of this position. Front-line nurse-managers perform the interesting and frustrating role of being the one in the middle. Management directives are received on the one hand, while, on the other hand, members of the unit who express needs for security, professional recognition, and independence, pressure their managers. The role is a difficult one indeed with a future forecast of more union intervention.

BIBLIOGRAPHY

Alexander, E. L. *Nursing Administration in the Hospital Care System*. St. Louis: C. V. Mosby, 1972.

Barnard, Chester I. *The Functions of the Executive*. Cambridge, Mass.: Harvard University Press, 1938.

Bennis, Warren G. "Leadership Theory and Administrative Behavior." *Administrative Science Quarterly* (December 1959): 259–301.

Davis, Keith. *Human Relations at Work*, 3rd ed. New York: McGraw-Hill, 1967.

Douglass, Laura Mae, and Bevis, Em Olivia. *Nursing Leadership in Action,* 2nd ed. St. Louis: C. V. Mosby, 1974.

"Florence Nightingale" in *Eminent Victorians,* Baltimore: Penguin Books, in association with Chatto and Windus Ltd. (London), 1948 (first published in 1918).

Fry, W. F., and Lauer, J. "The Planning Team: Why Include Nursing Leadership?" *Journal of Nursing Administration* (May 1972): 70–78.

Herzberg, Frederick. "One More Time: How Do You Motivate Employees?" *Harvard Business Review on Management*. New York: Harper & Row, 1975.

Koontz, Harold, and O'Donnell, Cyril. *Essentials of Management*. New York: McGraw-Hill, 1974.

Korman, Abraham K. "'Consideration,' 'Initiating Structure,' and Organizational Criteria—A Review." *Personnel Psychology,* vol. 19, no. 4 (Winter 1966): 361–379.

Korn, Thora. *Nursing Team Leadership,* 2nd ed. Philadelphia: Saunders, 1966.

Lewin, Kurt; Lippit, Ronald; and White, R. K. "Patterns of Aggressive Behavior in Experimentally Created Social Climates." *Journal of Social Psychology,* vol. 10, no 2 (May 1939): 271–299.

Likert, Rensis. *New Patterns of Management*. New York: McGraw-Hill, 1961.

Mann, F. C. "Toward an Understanding of the Leadership Role in Formal Organization." In *Leadership and Productivity,* edited by R. Dubin, G. Homan, and D. Miller. San Francisco: Chandler, 1964.

Maslow, Abraham. *Motivation and Personality*. New York: Harper, 1954.

McClelland, David C. *The Achieving Society*. Princeton, N.J.: D. Van Nostrand, 1961.

_____ and Burnham, David H. "Power Is the Great Motivator." *Harvard Business Review* (March–April 1976): 100–110.

McGregor, Douglas. *The Human Side of Enterprise*. New York: McGraw-Hill, 1960.

_____ . *Leadership and Motivation*. Cambridge, Mass.: M.I.T. Press, 1966.

Miller, D. I. "Leaders March to a Different Drummer," *Journal of Nursing Administration* (January–February 1971): 3.

Morse, John J., and Lorsch, Jay W. "Beyond Theory Y." *Harvard Business Review on Management*. New York: Harper & Row, 1975.

Rice, A. K. *The Enterprise and Its Environment*. London: Tavistock Publications, 1963.

Schlotfeld, Rozella. "Responsible Leadership: Whom for What?" *Nursing Science* (December 1963): 341.

Selznick, Philip. *Leadership in Administration*. Evanston, Ill.: Row-Peterson, 1957.

Tannenbaum, Robert, and Schmidt, Warren H. "How to Choose a Leadership Pattern." *Harvard Business Review* (March–April 1958): 95–101.

Taylor, Edwin K. "The Unsolved Riddle of Executive Success." *Personnel* (March–April 1960): 8–17.

Tead, Ordway. *The Art of Leadership*. New York: McGraw-Hill, 1935.

Chapter 14

Effective Performance Appraisal in Nursing

One of nurse-managers' major roles is the management of care-giving resources, including the evaluation of performance of the care-giving resources. Nurse-managers must be able on a periodic basis to assess performance of individuals who work on the unit. Many nurse-managers have viewed this responsibility with great apprehension because of the perceived confrontation that can result from providing feedback to an individual about his or her performance. These negative views need not be necessary if the appraisals are approached on a constant, objective basis in relation to position objectives.

Nurse-managers must approach this situation in a constructive way to help unit members toward greater improvement of performance for the organization and to help individuals satisfy their needs. Managers must remember that individuals have undergone reviews and evaluations throughout life, and they periodically want to know where they stand in terms of management's expectations.

PERFORMANCE APPRAISAL CONSIDERATIONS

In the past personnel evaluations were conducted on the basis of traits and personality, which presented the problems of favoritism. With the advent of management by objectives, a whole new era of appraisal of performance has come into being. Kellogg (1965) indicates that not only can organizations benefit from reviewing overall appraisal but that individuals can benefit from such a performance-appraisal process. The performance-appraisal process is more advantageous to the individual than other methods of evaluation because it provides a system of review that relates more closely to the position, is more objective in nature, has active and positive elements, is forward looking in orientation, and encourages the individual to accomplish objectives (Mali, 1975, p. 203).

In establishing an effective appraisal system, position descriptions must be well defined in the organizing process with verifiable objectives. The conceived objectives must be measurable in quantitative terms. They should be couched in terms of performance-oriented objectives that are reasonable and attainable within a specified period of time. As nurse-managers operate in a hospital setting, they are continually making informal appraisals of staff members. The cumulation of the appraisals comes to bear at the time of formal performance appraisal, when progress over a period of time is measured.

The position description as defined by verifiable objectives should be viewed in a dynamic sense. In the period of time between appraisals the actual tasks with a position may change because of changes in staff and technology, demands from administration and the medical staff, as well as external factors impinging on the operating environment. Before performing an appraisal, nurse-managers should ascertain that the position description is relevant to the role currently expected from the individual staff members. The appraisal will be based on the position description and, as a result, must accurately reflect what actually occurs in the unit. This function is often difficult to perform because managers may not be fully aware of the total role being performed by the employee in the unit. To uncover some of the deviations in role performance from the position description it is helpful to have the employee do a self-appraisal on an objective-by-objective basis with a final open-ended question related to other activities. This approach permits employees to examine what they have actually accomplished during the year. In this method, employees write reports of self-perceiving performance. A helpful format for this appraisal is to include three columns: one for objectives, one for self-appraisal, and one for the nurse-manager's comments. The purpose of the open-ended question is to cover activities performed but not included in the description. In addition, employees may often be hard-pressed to identify progress on one or two objectives. This occurrence usually indicates that the role has changed or that the employee has not accomplished what was delineated by the objective. The comparative function performed at this stage greatly assists in establishing that the appraisal is conducted on a relevant basis.

REWARD SYSTEMS

Following the establishment of functions, objectives, and their clustering into general descriptions for positions, the specifications of positions are determined. These specifications act as standards for personnel who will be hired to fill the created positions. The role expectations of the positions together with the specifications of the positions constitute a basis for establishing the general worth of the position, including a rating on a point basis of the experience and education required to perform the position. In an overall organizational sense, all positions should be rated. Once this rating has been completed, the ratings should be checked for accuracy and consistency in comparison with other positions. Next, an examination of current market pricing can be done to ensure that the pricing of positions is competitive with the prevailing market conditions in that job-market area. It is essential that similar positions at one institution are competitive in the job market with other institutions. When this research is accomplished and relative worth has been determined, the system can be tested for consistency among positions. At this point in time, the base pay has been determined for all positions at an entry level. The analysis of positions and their relative rating provide a rational basis for determining the base pay for positions.

Once the base-pay levels have been established, nurse-managers should examine the various variable pay mechanisms that can be used once a candidate has been hired for a position. In considering variable pay mechanisms that are available to nurse-managers, a general philosophy of variable pay must be stated. Many organizations have established a seniority system. This system is solely time-dependent and is not related to performance. Thus, as employees spend more time with an organization, the more they are rewarded, regardless of how well they have performed. Seniority has the obvious advantage of not requiring any review by management; it merely occurs with the passage of time. This form of variable pay encourages long service with the organization. Seniority has the definite advantage of providing security that assists in meeting lower level needs in Maslow's hierarchy. However, many younger personnel who are highly motivated find the seniority system stultifying. They feel that if they work hard and do a good job, they should progress at a faster pace in the organization than is permitted by the seniority system.

In lieu of a seniority system exclusively, many organizations have developed a merit system or merit/seniority system based on employee performance. The principal purpose of instituting a merit-oriented system is to recognize in the form of pay increases good performance rather than to encourage strictly longer service. The consideration of a merit system is not as simple as a seniority system and requires a greater amount of time on the part of nurse-managers to operate. Judgement of performance is the foundation upon which increases are determined. The performance-oriented appraisal provides feedback as a motivator for employees. These appraisals meet lower level needs by increasing compensation, but they also meet ego and self-esteem needs through positive reinforcement for a job well done.

There are some problems associated with this type of system. As with all evaluations, the measurement of progress can be a problem because the activities as performed do not necessarily lend themselves to measurement. Differences in perception of the appraiser can also create difficulties on an overall basis when the perceived performance of two employees is viewed as quite similar by them, whereas the appraisals of both demonstrate great divergence. Obviously, if some employees perform well and others do not, some employees will receive more than others, given limited funds available, possibly creating a negative atmosphere for those who did not fare well in the appraisal process.

Some organizations have developed a combination of seniority and performance-oriented increases. This system has obviously both the advantages and disadvantages of both systems. Many managers feel that it defeats the purpose of each system on an individual basis. This issue is certainly debatable.

More recently organizations have instituted a cost-of-living clause as part of the total reward system package. The cost-of-living factor is usually based on the consumer price index for a localized area. This aspect of reward is particularly germane during periods of high inflation in the economy. If this type of coverage is not provided, employees may personally not be as well off as they were a year earlier. Cost-of-living increases will barely maintain employee purchasing power. If the percentage of the increase is equal to the percentage of rising cost of living, employee income is merely keeping pace with already higher prices. In addition, with the graduated tax structure on personal incomes, even if the increase equals the cost-of-living percentage increase, the employee is in a higher tax bracket and actually has less disposable income. The best that one can expect is that the cost-of-living increase will merely be an attempt to keep the employee even with inflation.

Organizations provide other forms of compensation as part of the total reward system. These forms are usually referred to as supplementary compensation or fringe benefits. Included in this category are paid pension plans, health and accident insurance, and life insurance. In addition, the organization usually provides paid holidays, vacations, maternity leave, and continuing education activities. The examples given are only illustrative; the list varies from organization to organization and can be quite extensive in some cases.

If properly conceived of on a rational and consistent basis, the reward systems can act as a vehicle for rewarding performance and will assist individuals in meeting their needs. The degree to which higher level needs can be met by reward systems depends greatly on organizational philosophy and how much feedback is given to employees regarding their performance.

Recall that Herzberg (1968) developed two continuums of separate factors and labeled them "hygiene" and "motivators." Within those structures, salary and security were considered hygienic factors, whereas recognition and achievement were motivators. The implication is that money is not a motivator. However, money is often more than money (Patton, 1961). It can take many forms, and when related to performance, it can be a reflection of motivational factors. For example, if an organization uses a performance-oriented appraisal system, the additional money received by an employee actually represents recognition by management that a measure of achievement has been attained. The impact of reward for performance has been diluted because many managements attempt to maintain only marginal differences among employees' compensation and thereby minimize the actual effect of the recognition and achievement. In order for performance-appraisal systems to be effective, the reward systems must be based on creating more than marginal differences among employees in recognition of performance. Ideally, the reward system must perform a balancing act of recognition of individuals while providing mechanisms for stability and maintenance of the group (Drucker, 1973, p. 434).

APPRAISAL PROCESS

The performance-appraisal process is a part of the entire process of management. Management by objectives constitutes the forerunner and foundation for the appraisal process. This process represents an ongoing dynamic situation for nurse-managers. On a day-to-day basis nurse-managers are informally assessing the effectiveness of staff. Observations are made of staff and their interactions with other staff and with patients. Constructive comments are given to staff members to assist them in their performance on the unit. So appraisals are not quite as infrequent in occurrence as one might think.

Appraisal processes have changed over time. The traditional appraisal process was one couched in terms of employee characteristics, as previously mentioned. Under the traditional model, the manager did a scoring on characteristics and then gave criticism and praise to the employee. The employee played a very passive role in this approach. The manager's role was to tell employees where they stood in terms of these characteristics and more often than not had to sell the employee on the fact that the rating was correct (Maier, 1958, pp. 27–40).

The performance-appraisal system being suggested here is based on management by objectives. When the position description was originally developed, the employee participated in defining the objectives and standards of that position. Thus, when the time for performance appraisal occurs in a formal sense, nurse-managers review the employees' progress toward mutually agreed-upon objectives. It is the use of this behaviorally oriented approach that makes the performance appraisal interview much easier for managers than under the traditional model. The major element inherent in the traditional model has been removed—namely, confrontation. This does not mean that all possibilities of confrontation have been eliminated but rather significantly reduced.

Nurse-managers may have employees do self-appraisals as a phase of the appraisal process. Using this technique will often give employees an early-on view of their own performance before the interview and it helps to eliminate the possibility that the whole appraisal will be a surprise. It further helps in focusing on fewer issues because, in general, if the self-appraisal is valid in terms of measured performance then any perceived differences between the manager and the employee can be resolved.

As mentioned earlier it is important that the position description actually reflect the unit member's current responsibility. With this type of appraisal and approach, these areas not currently defined should become evident.

The interview itself is the most crucial aspect of the performance appraisal. Nurse-managers should view the interview not with apprehension but rather as an opportunity to assist members of the unit in carrying out assigned responsibilities. The orientation of a Theory-Y manager is strongly encouraged. The interview should be an opportunity for open dialogue that will result in definite feedback for employees and result in specific plans that are jointly determined to improve individual performance.

To conduct effectively an appraisal interview requires a certain amount of training. It is suggested that seminars be conducted by inservice departments for nurse-managers. These seminars can be most helpful to managers in gaining confidence and in fostering the appropriate positive attitudes for preparing for appraisal interviews. The use of role-playing among managers can be a most rewarding experience. It can identify negative statements that could significantly reduce the positive impact of the interview. Training for these interviews is certainly time well spent.

The behavioral approach to performance appraisals has certain limitations. As is true of the entire program of management by objectives, the performance-appraisal system as suggested takes more managerial and staff member time than does the more traditional approach. The objectives as delineated must also be measurable and reasonably attainable, or the entire basis of the appraisal will be subject to criticism. The behavioral approach seems to have considerable value with professional staff members but does not appear to be practical for more restricted and regimented jobs performed by other members of the unit. In these situations, it would appear more advisable to use a more traditional, structured format to achieve desired results in the review process. Some problems have also been encountered when the staffing pattern is such that the span of management or span of control becomes too large that a more structured approach appears necessary (Flippo, 1966, p. 261).

Thus, the performance-appraisal system has many complex aspects. It is not easy to administer but provides probably the greatest potential for assisting nurse-managers and individual employees in providing caregiving resources.

SUMMARY

A major role of nurse-managers is evaluation of performance of caregiving resources. The review of performance should be approached in a thoughtful and constructive manner and need not be considered in a negative way. Traditionally, appraisals were based on traits and personalities of individuals. Performance appraisals that are behaviorally oriented and based on a management-by-objectives system have the principal advantages of relating more closely to the position, of being more objective, of being more active and positive, of being forward-looking, and of encouraging the individual in the accomplishment of objectives.

Position descriptions are couched in verifiable objectives. The dynamic nature of position descriptions must be considered prior to appraisal. It is suggested that self-appraisal be incorporated as an interim step in the total appraisal process. This approach will assist managers in updating the position description and will orient employees for the appraisal.

Reward systems were examined including base-pay systems, variable-pay systems, and supplementary compensation systems. Base-pay systems must evolve from a logical, systematic process that is consistent among positions and is competitive with existing market conditions. Variable-pay systems include seniority and merit-rated aspects. The motivational aspects of merit-oriented systems were favored in lieu of seniority systems, which foster longevity and stability. Supplementary compensation systems included fringe benefits, such as pensions, life and health insurance in addition to paid holidays and vacations.

Money itself is not a motivator, but money is often a reflection of motivational factors.

Management by objectives is the foundation for the appraisal process. Appraisals are done informally by nurse-managers every day. Behaviorally oriented performance appraisal is designed so that employee progress is evaluated on mutually agreed-upon objectives that were developed by nurse-managers and individual employees. The confrontation aspects of more traditional approaches to performance appraisal can be minimized with behavioral orientation. Training sessions for conducting performance appraisals is recommended. The interview itself must be positive in nature, developing a plan for future improvement of performance.

The behavioral approach has certain limitations, including extensive use of time and measurement of performance; it does not appear to be a good appraisal method for routine jobs or when there is a wide span of management.

BIBLIOGRAPHY

Clissold, G. K., and Metz, E. A. "Evaluation—a Tangible Process." *Nursing Outlook* vol. 14, no. 3 (1977): 41–45.

Drucker, Peter F. *Management: Tasks, Responsibilities and Practices*. New York: Harper & Row, 1973.

Flippo, Edwin B. *Principles of Personnel Management*. New York: McGraw-Hill, 1966.

Herzberg, Frederick. "One More Time: How Do You Motivate Employees?" *Harvard Business Review*, vol. 46, no. 1 (January–February 1968).

Kellogg, Marion. *What to Do About Performance Appraisals*. New York: American Management Association, 1965.

Koontz, Harold. *Appraising Managers as Managers*. New York: McGraw-Hill, 1971.

Levinson, Harry. "Appraisal of what performance?" *Harvard Business Review*, vol. 54, no. 4 (July-August 1976): 30ff.

Mager, R. F., and Pipe, P. *Analyzing Performance Problems*. Belmont, Calif. Fearon, 1970.

Maier, Norman R. F. *The Appraisal Interview*. New York: Wiley, 1958.

Mali, Paul. *How to Manage By Objectives*. New York: Wiley, 1975.

Meyer, Herbert. "The Pay for Performance Dilemma". *Organizational Dynamics* (Winter 1975): 39–50.

Odiorne, George S. *Management by Objectives: A System of Managerial Leadership*. New York: Pitman, 1965.

Ortelt, J. "The Development of a Scale for Rating Clinical Performance." *Journal of Nursing Education,* vol. 5, no. 1 (1966): 15–17.

Patton, Arch. *Men, Money and Motivation*. New York: McGraw-Hill, 1961.

Rosen, A., and Abraham, G. E. "Evaluation of a Procedure for Assessing the Performance of Staff Nurses." *Nursing Research* 12. (Spring 1963): 78–82.

White, B. F., and Barnes, L. B. "Power Networks in the Appraisal Process." *Harvard Business Review,* vol. 49, no. 3 (May–June 1971): 101–109.

Chapter 15

Continuing Education in Nursing

As a nurse-manager, you have an important responsibility to the organization and to the individuals whom you supervise. This responsibility is continuing staff education. The impact of this responsibility transcends all operations in the unit. Certainly, individuals who join the unit bring with them various educational levels and backgrounds with necessary competencies in the delivery of nursing care to patients. Nurse-managers must provide opportunities for individual staff members' growth and development as well as inspiration for increased organizational effectiveness. The vehicle to assure these desired states is continuing education.

We shall examine the considerations that are essential for nurse managers to plan the appropriate types of continuing education opportunities for staff. The differences between education and training will be discussed as well as the probable sources of such opportunities. In addition, the level and extent of specialization has a definite bearing on this planning process, and these will be considered at some length.

INSERVICE EDUCATION

Every hospital setting has some form of inservice education available to its staff. Inservice departments in hospitals reflect the need of the organization to convey inhouse policies and procedures as they relate to the delivery of patient care. They tend to provide background to the individual employee with a heavy emphasis on the performance of one's position. The orientation of inservice education is basically that of training an individual to perform more in accordance with existing policies and procedures. Thus, in many cases the inservice department assists the individual to enhance skills.

The work of the inservice department is vital to the organization. It provides individuals with the opportunity of learning newer skills and permits a greater continuity in the way care is delivered to the patients. Individuals have an incentive to attend these sessions and to learn these skills because the more they are indoctrinated in the hospital's methods, the more their performance will be congruent with managerial expectations. Thus, the individual security is enhanced, assuring that the physiological needs will continue to be met. In addition, individual ego has a foundation of support through positive feedback from management and peers. Thus, inservice department training is important for all personnel, regardless of organization level or degree of specialization. However, among all the levels, training is more important for employees who operate at lower levels within the organization than for those in higher level positions.

EXTERNAL EDUCATION

Certainly, inservice education is valuable to all employees, including managers. However, for those employees who have a greater degree of formal education and experience, the need for professional growth and development can be only partially met by inservice efforts.

All registered nurses who work in the unit or department need external professional stimulation that transcends the available inservice programs. This fact is even more pronounced among the clinical nurse specialists. These external educational opportunities primarily come from the professional educational societies, which are principally nursing oriented. Opportunities of this nature generally consist of program content that has a more complex and in depth clinical basis than does the inservice educational opportunity. In addition, these programs permit exposure to nationally known teachers, clinicians, and colleagues from various parts of the country. Since exposure provides an intellectually stimulating experience that assists in the staff's professional development, it is important that nurse-managers plan and budget such external activities for professional staff members. The experiences are most valuable because they allow individuals to meet higher level needs through professional staff development.

As one looks again at Maslow's hierarchy of needs, it becomes readily apparent that inservice programs principally provide mechanisms for satisfaction of lower level needs, whereas the external education opportunities have the greatest potential for assisting the professional in meeting the higher level needs. Administration and the nursing office usually require nurse-managers to keep to a minimum the amount of staff days devoted to continuing education, for budgetary purposes. However, the need for continuing education opportunities is greatest among the most qualified members of staff. If staff turnover can be minimized, this is a reasonable bargaining position with administration for nurse-managers.

Many nurse-managers develop a feeling of concern that if the key people on the staff are exposed to many outside opportunities, staff may be attracted to other hospitals. If there are few opportunities available at the hospital, this could very well be the case. On the other hand, if there are a number of opportunities available to the staff, its members may act as good will ambassadors and may attract key people to the hospital. This approach can also be used as a bargaining tool with administration. It represents the trade-offs between staff needs, availability of funding, and organizational philosophy in support of continuing education for staff.

NATURE OF NURSE-MANAGER DEVELOPMENT

So far, we have considered continuing education needs of the staff. Now we shall look at some aspects of education and continuing education for the nurse-manager.

In the recent past, it was quite normal managerial practice in the hospital setting to "promote" a very good clinician to an administrative position. In an earlier chapter, we discussed the example of the effective bedside nurse being promoted to higher and higher administrative levels and responsibilities so that patient contact was virtually eliminated. At the same time the education basis of the nurse had been almost exclusively toward patient care, which is where it should be. However, in reality, shortly after graduation, a portion of the nursing graduates will be placed in positions of significant managerial responsibility.

Certainly, debate has gone on for years and will continue about the appropriate balance of theory and practice in nursing curricula. In spite of these continuing debates over clinical theory and clinical practice, more and more nursing faculties are recognizing that in actual practice, a good portion of graduates are being placed in managerial roles. For this reason, many nursing faculties have recommended that at least one course be devoted to leadership in nursing. This action represents a good first start toward the development of a more comprehensive course in management. As more and more faculties realize that leadership is only one part of directing, and directing is one part of management, there will be more movement toward courses in management for the nurses.

One of the real problems in curriculum development is whether management courses should be mandatory or voluntary. With the increasing pressure on the health care system to demonstrate increased effectiveness, it would seem that every nurse should have one course in management. This approach would permit nurses to manage resources better and would greatly assist managers by giving them a better understanding of the management process. Thus, greater staff support would be possible through greater understanding. For those nurses who have a special interest in management, perhaps a second course on an optional basis could be incorporated into the curriculum. This course could include Harvard-type case studies that could build on the first course, which most certainly must be heavily couched in management and organization theory. Ideally, for those nurses with a desire to continue their studies, a master's degree program in management could be provided for nurses. This course of study would provide in-depth opportunities to examine all management functions with particular emphasis on decision-making strategies.

To meet a more immediate need for nurses who are managers without the benefit of formal education in management, many organizations and professional societies have now made some limited continuing education programs available. This much-needed offering is available, and the number and complexity of these offerings are expected to continue. At last, a concerted effort is being made to meet this need.

Approaches to Nurse-Manager Development

As nurse-managers look ahead to professional development, it is helpful to be aware of the different approaches that have been used in manager development. The original foundation consists of a series of topics that address the formal functions of management—namely, planning, organizing, directing, and controlling. It is important to understand the framework of management as described in these approaches before advancing to other education approaches.

Once this foundation has been established, then it is most beneficial to examine approaches that address the behavioral science view of management. Behavioral science considers the humanistic aspect of management and how it will lie on the formal management structure and help bridge the gap from management theory to what one actually experiences in practice. These considerations permit nurse-managers to develop concern and understanding of individuals and groups that operate in the organizational environment.

The expansion of behaviorally oriented programs for managers has resulted in the T-groups or sensitivity training.

The T-group concept was initially conceived by Kurt Lewin and has been significantly expanded by the National Training Laboratories and the Human Relations Research Group at UCLA. These groups tend to be small and meet over a period of time. Sessions can be of short or long duration. Primary focus is for the group to observe the thoughts and feelings of members of the group. In addition, feedback is provided to the members that supposedly assists in contrasting their perceived self-images with their images as perceived by the group. The contrasted difference between individual and group hopefully can induce change. Ideally, the individual can eventually express suppressed feelings so that the group can assist the individual in dealing with these feelings in an open manner. From an organization standpoint, the T-group addresses subject matter that is not related to organizational purpose but is designed to assist individuals in dealing with self and others. Certainly, nurse-managers who do not possess a form of self-assurance cannot be expected to deal effectively with others. The success of T-groups has not been established. Allen (1973) has suggested this conclusion and indicates that "organization development" may have assumed some of the preeminence previously enjoyed by the T-group approach.

The major drawback of the T-group is its nonorganizational orientation. To overcome this negative aspect of T-groups and to make significant contributions to organizations, a newer approach was established, known as organizational development. Miner (1973) perceived that organization development occurred to make T-groups and other similar vehicles more relevant to management. The primary emphasis of organizational development is to secure change in management and an organization on a long-term basis. This approach is based on the premise that changes in the attitudes, motives, and values of individuals toward more participative management will assist in making organizational change.

Organizational development has come under considerable criticism because of its fragmented approach to change instead of a more comprehensive approach that would affect the total organization. In addition, it has received much criticism for its overemphasis on human needs in contrast to organizational needs, as well as its emphasis on behavior prior to diagnosis. The overall stress on the informal organization has also drawn issue from more traditionally oriented managers. The general behavioral approach of organizational development supports McGregor's Theory Y, and if carried through to completion, can result in significant demand for reorganization. Organizational development can produce changes in the organization that can greatly pressure its present existence. Therefore, many higher level managers may have more to lose by the changes than lower level participants. Evans (1974) recently reported on many organizational development programs that had not been successful.

The most recent approach to management development has come from the work of Luthans (1973). He describes a motivational approach to organizational behavior that he calls organization behavior modification. This approach attempts to implement organizational goals by using appropriate organizational stimuli to control behavior of individuals and to provide reinforcement mechanisms as reward systems for supportive behavior patterns. The vehicles proposed for use in the approach include money, responsibility, and social approval of behavior. Organization behavior modification is perhaps too new and untried to report significant studies of success or failure. It would appear that this approach is less threatening to management, but whether or not it provides sufficient opportunities for other staff members to participate in the decision-making process is unknown. Perhaps the development of this orientation toward behavior modification may indicate a shifting in managerial emphasis more toward a traditional school of management with implied manipulation/motivational basis to achieve desired results.

Regardless of the approaches to which nurse managers are exposed over time, all of these programs have positive aspects that can assist them in becoming more astutely aware of management problems. In many cases these problems provide mechanisms for coping with problems and for finding appropriate solutions.

Philosophy of Continuing Education

From a management standpoint, it is necessary that a philosophy be developed for continuing education of all staff. A definite commitment must be secured from top management before beginning the planning of continuing education programs for staff. This commitment can be expressed as a long-term goal and preferably should include short-term quantifiable objectives for the department of nursing and all units. For the specified goals and objectives to become reality, it is necessary to budget and fund these activities. Once management has provided the overall mechanisms to make continuing education a fact of organizational life, it must be stated at the outset that the major type of development has to come from the individual on the unit and in the department. Thus, self-development and the motivation for development are essential for any continuing education program to be successful. Staff members cannot be forced to attend inservice programs or external educational programs and made to learn. The drive and desire to learn must come from the individual.

Nurse-managers have an obligation to set an environmental tone of exchange of ideas and openness that will permit the individuals to be in continuous learning situations. All too often individuals work in unit environments that have stultified learning because of the heavy authoritarian approach used by managers. Nurse-managers orientation that builds on Theory Y management will foster a more open working environment and stimulate the members of the unit.

The orientation of staff toward the continuing education opportunities is also necessary to help assure the success of the experience. The members of the unit or department should not view continuing education solely as the number of hours, number of CEUs (Continuing Education Units), or number of courses to be completed. The essential thrust of continuing education must be development and change of the individual. Through knowledge and skills obtained, the individual should gain greater self-assurance and hopefully be able to bring to bear some of the changes for the betterment of patient care and more efficient use of resources.

Nurse-managers must prepare a plan for continuing education of staff. At the outset, it is readily recognized that needs vary among staff depending on education, experience, and responsibilities. Therefore, nurse-managers should make sure that inservice programs are available and that the staff attends those appropriate to the needs of individuals and the organization. In the case of highly educated specialists, a greater exposure to externally available programs should be included in the planning of continuing education. A series of continuing education experiences should also be planned for nurse-managers to permit a basis for maintaining currency as well as providing a periodic intellectual stimulation.

The planning of these educational opportunities is an ongoing responsibility of management. Given the nature and speed of changes occurring in nursing in particular to health care in general, all that one can hope for is to stay abreast of current developments.

EVALUATION OF CONTINUING EDUCATION

At one time continuing education was though of as a nice supplement. However, with the development of the complexities of society and health care, continuing education is generally viewed as being voluntary.

With the increased demands of society for better health care and the involvement of the federal government in providing mechanisms for quality review, the needs for both inservice and external education programs have greatly increased. Much pressure is now being placed on administration and the nursing office to make sure that conformance with newly enacted legislation is a reality. The increasing complexity of medical and nursing care has also resulted in a great proliferation of programs to meet the needs of keeping up with these new developments. In some cases, the developments are occurring at such a rapid pace that new graduates have reported that the new developments had not been included in their curricula.

At this time, nursing is at a critical stage with regard to continuing education. A few states make it mandatory for relicensing, and many are considering making it mandatory. Concomitantly, hospital administrations have been placed in the difficult position of trying to contain spiraling costs of health care while making more funds available for continuing education.

So, nurse-managers are facing the situation in which staff demands for continuing education are proliferating while the funds to support these much-needed activities are becoming less available. Thus, the mandate is becoming quite clear. Nurse-managers must demonstrate that the programs for continuing education are needed and are cost effective. In other words, the organization is more likely to support programs in which the organization can see some future benefits. This justification can probably be best accomplished by securing additional benefits from these programs, particularly in the case of external programs by having staff members who attend these sessions provide inhouse or inservice classes based at least partially on these programs.

It is most ironic in an era when continuing education has come into its own that the funds to support these activities seem to be less available on a per-capita basis.

SUMMARY

The nurse-manager's role in continuing education is important and the impact of this responsibility transcends all operations. Individual staff needs for growth and development as well as for increased organizational effectiveness can be met by continuing education.

Training is generally provided by inservice departments and tends to emphasize enhancement of skills that usually relate to existing organizational policies and procedures. This training is oriented toward improving individual performance and conforming to organizational needs. Such training assists the individual in meeting the lower level needs of Maslow's hierarchy of needs. Training tends to be relatively more important for individuals lower in the organizational hierarchy.

In contrast to training, education tends to be more general in providing growth and development for the professional. These programs are usually available through external educational sources, such as professional nursing societies. Educational programs offered through these mechanisms tend to meet higher level needs of individual staff members primarily because of the exposure to nationally known teachers and practitioners as well as colleagues from various parts of the country.

Nurse-managers also need continuing education. Initially, it is assumed that managers have had at least one course in formal management theory as well as a Harvard-type case-study course for practice as part of their formal education. For managers without benefit of formal education in management, many organizations have programs available to meet this need.

There are many approaches that have been used to assist in manager development. These approaches include formal management theory, general behavioral management theory, T-group or sensitivity training, organizational development and organization behavior modification.

It is necessary that each organization develop a philosophy of continuing education. Goals and objectives should be defined and implemented with appropriate budgetary and funding provisions. Concomitantly, the major type of development must come from the individual on the unit or department. Self-development and motivation for development are the key underlying foundations for the success of any continuing education program. Continuing education should be viewed as a growth and development opportunity rather than merely as the accumulation of hours, CEUs, or courses.

Nurse-managers must develop a plan for continuing education for members of departments or units. Appropriate planning incorporates differences in education, experiences, and organizational needs in establishing any program for continuing education.

Given the increased demand for more continuing education and the shrinking availability of funding, it is imperative that nurse-managers establish the justification for attendance as well as the cost effectiveness in organizational terms particularly for attendance at outside education programs.

BIBLIOGRAPHY

Allen, L. A. "The T-Group: Short Cut or Short Circuit?" *Business Horizons,* vol. 16, no. 4 (August 1973): 53–64.

Evans, M. G. "Failures in OD Programs: What Went Wrong?" *Business Horizons,* vol. 17, no. 2 (April 1974): 18–22.

Luthans, F. *Organizational Behavior.* New York: McGraw-Hill, 1973.

Miner, J. B. "The OD-Management Development Conflict." *Business Horizons,* vol. 16, no. 6 (December 1973): 33.

National Training Laboratory in Group Development. *Explorations in Human Relations Training: An Assessment of Experience, 1947–1953.* Washington, D.C.: National Education Association, 1953.

Chapter 16

The Involvement
Process in Nursing

Chris Argyris (1964, p. 59) hypothesized "that the more rigidity, specialization, tight control, and directive leadership the worker experiences, the more he will tend to create antagonistic adaptive activities." As a result of these management-imposed conditions, the individual will most likely exhibit various forms of adaptive behavior including absenteeism, resignation, aggression, and requests for additional compensation to combat working conditions (Argyris, 1964, pp. 60–63).

Many nurse-managers can easily cite various situations in the unit environment that may cause adaptive behavior by unit personnel. Probably one of the hardest incidents for individuals on the unit has been when the nurse-manager announces a change in organization policy or procedure and provides no rationale for the change. When members of the unit ask why, they are simply told that "administration has decided that it would be done that way." How can employees feel committed to implement the change? How committed do they feel when they have not been involved or even consulted about a change that will, in fact, change the way they do their jobs? It seems to be human nature that people do not want to be told what to do without some degree of involvement in the decision-making process. Such instances make individuals feel that they do not really count and that they can be easily exchanged by another interchangeable personnel unit. Thus, staff quickly loses any feeling of self-worth. As a result, they begin feeling a sense of alienation toward the unit and the organization since they have virtually no influence on what is happening. Many times a condition of powerlessness and helplessness comes over the individual (Dean, 1961).

These questions will now be examined in terms of motivation, involvement, and morale. These behavioral influences are most important to the effective operation of the nursing unit and department. Without a motivational base, employees have essentially no real incentive to perform.

MOTIVATIONAL BASES

In order to motivate employees on the unit, it is necessary that a conducive environment be established. Motivation is derived from motive or the "inner state that energizes, activates or moves and that directs or channels behavior towards goals" (Berelson & Steiner, 1964, p. 246). We know from the work of Maslow (1954) that basic human needs fit into a hierarchy. They are usually considered as expressed wants that have not yet been satisfied. Thus, an individual who has unsatisfied needs wants to satisfy those needs under the appropriate conditions. In a work situation, such conditions are primarily set by management.

As we examined the work of Herzberg (1959, 1968) and others, we noted that a two-factor theory of motivation existed among workers. Some factors were not motivators (hygiene factors), whereas other factors were motivators. This latter group was found to be motivators primarily because they had the ability to produce satisfaction, whereas the former factors could not. The motivators related to job-content factors. In other words, such work-related factors as recognition, advancement, growth in responsibility, achievement, and challenging work constituted the foundation for worker motivation. Research established that the hygiene factors of salary, job security, working conditions, and so forth are usually provided to most workers. The lack of these factors did not produce satisfaction, but their lack produced dissatisfaction. It is apparent that the motivational factors must be examined with great vigor to improve the effectiveness of the unit. How can nurse-managers increase the conduciveness of the unit environment to enhance individual opportunity for recognition, advancement, growth in responsibility, achievement, and the overall challenge of the work to be performed?

INVOLVEMENT AND INFLUENCE

The behaviorists in management have stressed the concept that motivation of employees can be accomplished by permitting them to have an influence on their working environment through involvement in the decision-making process (McGregor, 1960). Various concepts in management are used to implement the ideas of influence and involvement of employees. When employees are given the opportunity of "becoming involved," they will invest time and effort, as well as emotion, to improving the effectiveness of the unit and organization.

Before embarking on the approaches that can be used in the involvement process, there are certain managerial considerations that nurse-managers must take into account. First, what possible impact does the involvement of others in the management decision process have on the authority and power of the nurse-manager? Many nurse-managers are apprehensive about this process because they feel that "they may lose control of the situation." Some nurse-managers have stated that they cannot permit such involvement because "others" will take over their jobs and control of their units. These nurse-managers reflect a more traditional management approach, which strongly resists any input from unit personnel. To a certain degree these managers tend to be insecure. Remember that leadership can only occur when followership is a reality. Without such followership, the leader can be ineffective and even powerless. The fact that a command is uttered by the nurse-manager, in a traditional management sense, is no guarantee that the command will actually be followed. In today's society nurse-managers should be astutely aware that members of the unit tend to be better educated. Thus, people do not generally accept a command in a blind fashion but will tend to question assumptions much more frequently than has been true in the past. For these reasons, nurse-managers must strongly consider the active involvement of many members of the unit.

There are advantages in increasing influence and involvement of employees for the overall effectiveness of the unit or department. When individuals are involved in the decision-making process, they become emotionally involved and, in many cases, are committed to the resulting decision. This effect means that employees will, in general, work diligently to make sure that the decision is implemented. This active commitment can result in good employee performance, which requires less supervision and, in fact, demonstrates elements of self-control over assigned responsibilities. This commitment often produces increased productivity (Likert, 1961, p.119). In a health-care and nursing environment, such increased productivity has the effect of adding new staff without actually adding new staff. In a nursing environment, it is generally felt that increased staff can produce increased quality of nursing care. If existing staff can be sufficiently motivated to increase productivity, the developed productivity produces an in-kind type staff increase and should increase the quality of nursing care delivered to patients. Given this premise, the quality of care should be enhanced, whereas the cost of care to patients would not be proportionately increased.

With possible increased productivity and quality of care comes an increased morale for members of the unit. When employees are actively involved in the managerial decision-making process, a greater acceptance of decisions is likely to occur. It should be emphasized that involvement does not necessarily mean that the final decision by nurse-managers conforms to the input and recommendations of the staff members on the unit. The primary concept is that the input and suggestions of staff are seriously considered by management. It is quite surprising how often the suggestions of staff are not even considered! Whoever thought that the ideas of one person might be superior to the ideas of two or three or more? Such employee involvement has a positive effect on absenteeism and turnover. The general attitudes of staff are also more positive, which results in fewer complaints and in a staff that is much more amenable to change.

Should all staff members at all levels be involved in the managerial process? The answer must be diplomatic depending on the qualifications and experience of staff. However, in general, the answer must be no; not all individuals should be involved in the managerial decision-making process.

What criteria should be used to ascertain which members of the unit should be involved? Multiple criteria are needed. Certainly, the employee must have the interest and ability to become involved. Without such interest nurse-managers are wasting their time. When involvement is being contemplated, management must remember that the length of time for the decision-making process to occur has of necessity been lengthened. So interest and ability must be present. Employees must also have an attitude conducive to accepting the responsibility imposed by this expanded role. Unit members should be able to communicate ideas effectively. At the same time, nurse-managers must have positive feelings toward unit members so that proposed ideas and suggestions will be considered on their merit. If employees sense that managers are only going through the motions of the involvement process without serious commitment to it, they will probably not make a serious effort to become actively involved. Thus, it is imperative that there be trust between nurse-managers and employees, which represents the true binding force of an effective and meaningful involvement experience.

McClelland (1953, 1955, 1961, 1965), McClelland and Winter (1969), and McClelland and Burnham (1976) have done considerable research into the needs of individuals. These needs act as motivators, and the conditions for satisfying these needs can be enhanced through the involvement process. The needs identified by McClelland represent higher level needs in the Maslow hierarchy and to a great extent identify with Herzberg's motivation factor continuum. McClelland has called the three motivating needs or drives power, affiliation, and achievement. Generally, individuals with the need for power have to exert greater influence and control on their environments. The involvement process, when appropriately used, will permit individuals to exercise more influence on the environment through suggestions or ideas. Such involvement allows unit members to perceive a greater degree of control over the environment because of their input to changes that will likely occur in the unit. Most individuals have needs of acceptance by their fellow workers as evidenced by the social group they comprise. Involvement by unit members assists in the interaction with others and, by inclusion in the group itself, acts as a form of social acceptance. Thus, such involvement is a positive factor in permitting at least some satisfaction of the individual's need for acceptance. In the need for achievement, the individual must be challenged and likes to assume responsibility. By involving employees in the decision-making process, nurse-managers provide a vehicle to challenge them by exposing them to management problems and by suggesting possible avenues for resolution of such problems. In addition, employees have the opportunity to assume more responsibility for assisting management in tackling problems and seeking feasible solutions. Koontz and O'Donnell (1976, p. 576) state that "as a consequence, the right kind of participation yields both motivation and knowledge valuable for enterprise success." Therefore, nurse-managers should give serious consideration to actively pursuing employee involvement.

INVOLVEMENT IMPACT ON POSITIONS

We have examined the concept of job or position enlargement. Under this concept a concerted effort is made to make positions more interesting for employees. This enlargement process consists of taking dull, repetitive activities and incorporating more varied duties. A related but somewhat different concept is that of job or position enrichment. Enrichment is heavily based on the involvement process. The enrichment process attempts to stress the need to make positions not only more interesting but, more importantly, seeks to make them more challenging for the unit members. Enrichment of positions builds on the motivation research of Herzberg (1959, 1968). The enrichment concept then acts as the implementation mechanism for Herzberg's theory. To make positions more challenging, managers must emphasize the factors that relate to the motivational continuum. Thus, factors that identify with the content of positions should be examined carefully for possible enrichment. Specific factors to be addressed would include recognition, responsibility, and achievement.

The beginning of the process of enrichment usually starts with designing the position to allow for more variety of responsibility (using the enlargement concept). Next, the environment of the unit should be made conducive for enrichment. Nurse-managers must permit and encourage the involvement of unit members in the decision-making process. Unit members should be given more freedom in deciding how aspects of their positions may be executed. Where possible, the unit members should also be given responsibility for establishing the sequencing of work to be performed on the unit. Certain operating constraints are usually related to conditions of patients on the unit, which impose certain priorities of activities. These activities and their sequencing are not discretionary in nature and are system-imposed. However, other activities are somewhat discretionary, at least in terms of sequencing and application, which represent an area for freedom of decision making by the unit members. In addition, the involvement process can assist individual unit members to see better how their activities and responsibilities interface with other members of the unit. This element of the position-enrichment process helps the unit members understand more of the total process as well as the significant part they play in that process. By seeing the total picture through involvement and discussion, employees feel greater identification with the process and the other members who comprise the rest of the process.

Most of the applications of position enrichment have occurred in business. A rather complete analysis of the concept is contained in a book by Turner and Lawrence (1965). Varying degrees of success have been noted in many organizations. Fein (1974) reports that many organizations which have implemented enrichment programs found that nonmanagerial employees did not, in general, want more meaningful and challenging work. The acceptance and success of enrichment programs seem the greatest among management and professional employees. Fein's conclusions tend to support earlier works, which had questioned the universality of Maslow's hierarchy-of-needs concept. Do the hierarchy-of-needs concepts apply equally to all organization levels? Strauss (1963) concluded that a broad range of employees is not seeking higher level needs such as self-actualization. This conclusion would imply that the involvement process and position enrichment should be applied, as previously indicated, on a selective basis with interest and ability being the main considerations. Argyris (1960, Chapter 5) had identified that it was possible to have a stable work situation for employees in spite of the fact that they perform routine and programmed jobs. The implication seems apparent that even though these employees are not being motivated through the Herzberg-identified factors, they still seem to exhibit no active dissatisfaction, which runs contrary to the theory.

Thus, it would appear that position enrichment has certain selective uses. Members of the unit with established skills and professionals constitute the primary personnel market for possible position enrichment. Granted, their positions are more of a challenge than are positions requiring lower level skills. This does not mean that significant redesigning could not be done to enhance the challenge of those positions through appropriate enrichment processes.

The approach to developing an enrichment process should be one that is not strictly imposed by management. As is true with the entire involvement process, employees should be an integral part in the enrichment process. Employees must express interest and desire to want such enrichment to occur. Nurse-managers cannot overlook the great impact of a consultation with members of the unit, prior to implementation, by securing active commitment from those individuals who will be affected by enrichment.

Therefore, selectively used enrichment can provide a motivational basis for employees. It is a logical and necessary outgrowth of any involvement process if it is administered in an appropriate manner.

INVOLVEMENT AND ORGANIZATIONAL ENVIRONMENT

To design and develop an effective involvement system, nurse-managers must establish an organizational environment that will foster participation. First, managers should develop a philosophical orientation toward human behavior in accordance with Theory Y espoused by McGregor. Basically, Theory Y assumes that people have an intrinsic interest in their work, are self-motivated, are self-directed, and seek responsibility. Without a positive view of people, the exercise of involving people will be just that—an exercise. It is important that a behavioral approach be used in the organizing phase. In order for individuals to be motivated, the structure of the organization cannot be rigid. The span of management should be wide, thereby reducing the amount of direct supervision that is provided to employees. The amount of direct control over activities should be reduced permitting the evolution of more self-control. Positions should be developed with some input from members of the unit. Opportunities should be made available for diversification in responsibilities of position. Nurse-managers must be careful not to overengineer positions so that there is extreme overspecialization. Thus, the structuring of roles and positions on a more diversified basis can promote individual freedom and initiative without producing a threat to the individual's ego.

In the same vein, nursing management must develop appropriate mechanisms that will permit flexibility for the fusion of individual differences into the environment. This type of accommodation gives unit members a feeling of fitting in with the unit and the organization. This best-fit type of approach appears to develop a competence motivation in unit members and is most relevant in developing an effective nursing unit.

Building on the work of McClelland, Litwin and Stringer (1968) conducted research on what they defined as organizational climate. In testing the concepts of power, affiliation, and achievement, they found that the more structured an organization, the greater the need for power. The needs for affiliation and achievement were lower the more structured the organization. Thus, to increase an individual's drive for achievement and affiliation, a less tightly structured environment would appear to be necessary. Litwin's and Stringer's results only partially supported this contention. In organizations in which responsibility was high, a stronger relationship existed between achievement and responsibility, but little relationship existed between responsibility and affiliation. Their research does present strong evidence that the environment created for employees will, to a large extent, determine the amount of motivation an individual will exhibit with regard to achievement.

To implement an involvement system effectively some additional mechanisms are necessary in developing the environment. On an informal and daily basis, it is necessary that a consultative attitude pervade the nursing unit. This tone should be set by nurse-managers. The continual interactions among colleagues seeking consultative advice is a way to ensure that the prevailing atmosphere in the unit is conducive for involvement. On a more formal basis, weekly meetings to discuss current developments and to seek input from unit members will do much to encourage unit members to contribute ideas and observations. In addition, this type of vehicle is helpful in keeping every member informed of developments before they become a reality. The prescheduling of these meetings will create a situation in which members of the unit will be collecting observations and ideas for sharing with others on a consultative basis during the week. This type of formal and informal consultation fosters a feeling of joint responsibility and thereby assists in the unit members' sharing the concern and welfare of the unit and the organization.

SUMMARY

People do not want to be told what to do without some degree of involvement in decisions that will affect how they execute their duties. If they are not involved, they will develop various antagonistic adaptive behaviors. In addition, they have a feeling of powerlessness because they have no influence on what is happening.

Motivation is basically an individual inner state that is activated and directs behavior toward the achievement of goals. The individual's unsatisfied needs are thought to be the driving force that activates and directs behavior. Research has indicated that certain factors related to job content tend to act as motivators. These factors include recognition, advancement, growth in responsibility, achievement, and challenging work.

Behaviorists have suggested that motivation can be secured by permitting individuals to be involved in the decision-making process. Employees who are involved demonstrate an investment of time, effort, and emotion to the process and thereby develop an increased commitment and greater understanding.

Increasing an employee's influence and involvement can produce increased productivity and morale. With increased productivity, it is hypothesized that quality of nursing care should increase due to the in-kind staff increase impact.

Involvement should be accomplished according to criteria. Interest and ability are essential for such involvement by employees. Trust must also be evident between nurse-managers and employees.

The concepts of achievement, affiliation, and power were identified as employee motivators. The involvement process can assist unit members in moving toward the satisfaction of these needs.

The impact of the involvement process on positions can produce a situation of position enlargement and enrichment. The enrichment concept attempts to make positions challenging for individuals. Factors to be considered for possible enrichment include recognition, responsibility, and achievement. The acceptance and success of enrichment programs has been the greatest among management and professional employees. Other employees do not, in general, want more meaningful or challenging work.

Organizational environment is important in securing a conducive situation for an effective involvement system. Research has shown that the environment created for employees will tend to determine the amount of motivation an individual will have. Nurse-managers must provide the necessary environmental conditions by fostering a consultative attitude and atmosphere in the nursing unit.

BIBLIOGRAPHY

Argyris, Chris. *Understanding Human Behavior*. Homewood, Ill.: Irwin, 1960.
_____. *Integrating the Individual and the Organization*. New York: Wiley, 1964.
Berelson, Bernard, and Steiner, Gary A. *Human Behavior: An Inventory of Scientific Findings*. New York: Harcourt, Brace and World, 1964.

Dean, Dwight C. "Alienation: Its Meaning and Measurement." *American Sociological Review* 26 (October 1961); 753–758.

Fein, Mitchell. "Job Enrichment: A Reevaluation." *Sloan Management Review*, vol. 15, no. 2 (Winter 1974): 69–88.

Herzberg, F. "One More Time: How Do You Motivate Employees?" *Harvard Business Review*, vol. 46, no. 1 (January–February 1968).

_____; Mauser, B.; and Synderman, B. *The Motivation to Work*. New York: Wiley, 1959.

Koontz, Harold, and O'Donnell, Cyril. *Management: A Systems and Contingency Analysis of Managerial Functions*, 6th ed. New York: McGraw-Hill, 1976.

Likert, Rensis. *New Patterns of Management*. New York: McGraw-Hill, 1961.

Litwin, G. H., and Stringer, R. A., Jr. *Motivation and Organizational Climate*. Cambridge, Mass.: Harvard Graduate School of Business Administration, 1968.

Maslow, Abraham. *Motivation and Personality*. New York: Harper, 1954.

McClelland, David C. *The Achievement Motive*. New York: Appleton-Century-Crofts, 1953.

_____. *Studies in Motivation*. New York: Appleton-Century-Crofts, 1955.

_____. *The Achieving Society*. Princeton, N.J.: D. Van Nostrand, 1961.

_____. "Achievement Motivation Can Be Developed." *Harvard Business Review, vol. 43, no. 1 (January–*February 1965): 6–24.

_____, and Burnham, David H. "Power Is the Great Motivator." *Harvard Business Review,* vol. 54, no. 2 (March–April 1976): 100–110.

_____ and Winter, David G. *Motivating Economic Achievement*. New York: The Free Press, 1969.

McGregor, Douglas. *The Human Side of Enterprise*. New York: McGraw-Hill, 1960.

Strauss, George. "The Personality vs. Organization Theory." In *Individualism and Big Business*, edited by Leonard Sayles. New York: McGraw-Hill, 1963.

Turner, A. N., and Lawrence, P. R. *Industrial Jobs and the Worker*. Cambridge, Mass.: Harvard Graduate School of Business Administration, 1965.

Chapter 17

The Communication
Process in Nursing

Koontz and O'Donnell (1976, p. 610) state that "it is no exaggeration to say that communication is the means by which organized activity is unified." Communication is central to the nurse manager's role. "There is simply no way communication skills can be separated from leadership abilities because the most usual mode of exercising leadership is through the interactive process, which uses communicating as a primary vehicle" (Douglass and Bevis, 1974, p. 60).

Communication is usually taken for granted. Nurse-managers often believe that by the mere utterance of directives they are communicating and that members of the unit receive and fully understand the communications. The receiver of the communication is then expected to take the intended necessary action. Inappropriate action provides feedback to managers that something has gone wrong. This type of situation occurs too often in nursing units throughout the country. It is necessary that we examine the components of communication and the communication process to increase our understanding of how communication works and how nurse-managers can effectively improve their leadership. Tannenbaum,

Weschler, and Massarik (1961, p. 24) feel so strongly about the role of communications in leadership that they define leadership in that sense as "interpersonal influence, exercised in situation and directed, through the communication process, toward the attainment of a specified goal or goals."

COMPONENTS OF COMMUNICATION AND EFFECTIVENESS

Before we can analyze problems in communication, we must first examine the components of communication. Most discussions about communication begin with the sender and what content he or she intends to convey. Then they discuss the receiver and how validation or nonvalidation of the communication occurs. Basically, when a communication is received and interpreted it becomes known as a message, subject to clarification and possible modification through feedback to the sender. The sender proceeds to send a clarification to make sure that the intent of content is received and interpreted by the receiver. This process of communication can continue until an understanding of thoughts is conveyed from one mind to another. The process has a circular nature. However, I contend that too much initial emphasis is on the sender and the context of the communication to be sent to the receiver. I do not mean to imply that these aspects are not important, but rather to make communications more effective, the fewer iterations required to secure understanding, the more effective the communication. Certainly, when a nurse-manager has "a message to send," he or she ought to consider the rough content and proposed medium from the point of view of the receiver before finalizing them. Considering receiver orientation medium from the point of view of the receiver orientation before conveying a communication is perhaps one of the most neglected areas in communication.

If nurse-managers work to anticipate how a thought might be received, given the orientation and background of the potential receiver, there can be a greater meeting of minds. Anticipation and emphasis on receptivity need to be stressed by managers. Preliminary work of this nature can result in a reorientation of the initial approach to be used, as well as a couching of the content to improve the acceptance to the receiver.

In some situations nurse-managers approach a member of the unit with content that resulted from considerable thought and previous discussion with others. Following such extensive thought, managers are fully oriented to the content, and when it is conveyed to unit members, the content and rationale often do not mesh. Nurse-managers provide only the core of thought without benefit of background and process leading to the final communication provided to the receiver. This frequent situation occurs because the sender and receiver do not have the same background information. Thus, the receiver cannot be expected to respond on the same level of discussion as the sender. It is only through feedback, modification, and clarification that the sender and receiver can attempt to approach the same level of information and understanding. Thus, it is necessary that a receiver orientation be practiced by the sender to enhance the effectiveness of communications.

RESPONSIBILITY AND ACCOUNTABILITY

We have stressed the receiver-oriented role of the nurse-manager as sender. However, the burden of responsibility for communications cannot rest only with managers. The responsibility for communications is the shared responsibility of all members of the unit, department, and hospital. Nurse-managers have important roles in sending clear, concise, and understandable communications. Unit members also have the responsibility to listen and to try to understand what is being conveyed and to take appropriate action. Furthermore, when the unit member is the sender responsibility lies with the unit member, and the nurse-manager must listen attentively and seek understanding.

The responsibilities are clear depending on the situation. In working in a patient-care environment where a vast majority of communications are occurring for the purpose of affecting change in the care of patients, the responsibility for communications is paramount. If nurse-managers do not clearly and understandably communicate a directive, the resulting patient care may be given inappropriately. Similarly, when a unit member observes certain developments in a patient's conditions and conveys them to the nurse-manager who does not fully listen, the resulting advice may not be in the best interest of the patient. Thus, the accountability for effective communications in the unit and department cannot be overemphasized. In extreme cases, if the patient does not receive the expected care, given the condition of the patient, possible legal action may be taken by the patient and/or family. With the ever-increasing emphasis on responsibility and accountability in the delivery of nursing care to patients, the mandate is clear—if a communication is not fully understood, ask. It is your responsibility to do so, and if you do not, you may be held accountable for inappropriate care.

FORMAL AND INFORMAL INFORMATION SYSTEMS

Thus far, we have examined the development of the formal organization, which included a hierarchy of levels within the organization. The formal hierarchy constitutes what is called the formal organization, with defined responsibilities at each level and a delegation of formal authority in the structure.

As the lines of authority are conceived, lines of communication coincide with the formal lines of authority. These lines of communication comprise the formal channels of communication. This type of channel is used by nurse-managers regardless of leadership style. Managers view this channel as the vehicle to disseminate orders and directives to unit members. The flow of information through this channel is usually referred to as downward communication implying that it is following the authority structure from top to bottom. Communication through this structure can take on various forms from a chain of command (face-to-face or written), hospital newsletters, policy and procedures manuals, letters and payroll envelope stuffers, and so on.

The more traditional nurse-manager will use downward channels almost exclusively, whereas more behaviorally oriented nurse managers will use these channels to a lesser degree. Managers practicing a more behavioral approach will seek ideas and input from unit members in a consultation, stressing the need for member involvement. In these cases nurse-managers foster the development of channels from the unit members to the nurse-manager. The flow of information and ideas is basically up the hierarchical structure and is usually referred to as upward communication. This type of communication occurs in all organizations regardless of leadership style being practiced by management. However, the leadership style greatly determines the use of the system. The more traditional nurse manager primarily views upward communication as the feedback portion of the communication process. In contrast, the behaviorally oriented managers will use it for feedback but will greatly encourage its use for the initiation of sending new communications from members of the unit. Encouraging the upward flow of ideas through the involvement process greatly assists unit members in feeling more a part of the total management process, and increases productivity and morale. Communication through this channel takes various forms: chain of command in reverse, consultation, grievance and complaints, input from labor unions (e.g., ANA). The upward flow of communications is usually referred to as the informal system, even though some of the forms have been established by management. For the purpose of our discussion, we shall consider them informal, since management technically does not generally initiate the sending of communications up the organization unless so required as feedback to inquiries by higher level management. This condition tends to be less true if higher management has a behavioral orientation.

It has been generally established that when nursing management uses the downward flow of information, a considerable amount of time is consumed going through all of the organizational levels. In all organizations, employees establish what is known as a grapevine. This process of passing the word is a most effective system in terms of time, although sometimes the message being conveyed may get distorted. The speed of this process is rather astounding to management. For this reason, many hospitals have instituted a lateral information flow, which permits almost everyone to receive the communication at about the same time. It can be quite embarrassing for managers to find out about new developments through employees and the grapevine before receiving it formally from the nursing office or administration. In addition, it is important to remember that information is power, and those who possess the information have gained power through its acquisition.

MESSAGE CONSIDERATIONS

Nurse-managers must develop expertise regarding the basic vehicle to be used in sending a message. Whether it is written or oral depends on certain considerations. Certainly, if there will be a need for documentation, the message must be written. If the content is required for legal purposes or possible future legal purposes, it should be written. Obviously then, written communication is the preferred vehicle if records have to be kept for whatever reason. In a written form, messages then need to be more thoughtfully developed. This fact can easily be seen by dictating into a tape recorder and having the dictation typed as compared to formally writing the message on paper. The level and complexity of the dictated message should be less than the written message. This differential can be minimized with practice.

The written message will initially take more time than the oral message and will be more expensive to produce. However, if the original message has not been carefully composed, then it may in fact foster a series of messages as feedback for clarification which could actually cost the hospital considerably more in both time and expense. Oral communication is faster initially and provides the opportunity for immediate feedback for clarification. Many nurse managers have used a combination of oral and written for the same situation and have used them in concert with one another. In this situation nurse managers convey messages orally, receive immediate feedback and clarification, and then send out written memoranda confirming the oral discussion. This approach can have the advantage of speed, feedback, clarification, and it produces a record. In addition, unit members can implement the suggested change while the confirming portion is in process.

There are time and cost considerations in using both written and oral vehicles for messages. For example, a letter or memorandum can cost anywhere from $5 to $15, depending on length, complexity, cost of support personnel, and the amount of reproduction required. Included in the cost is the time taken by the manager to initially compose and later to review before signing the letter. On the other hand, oral communication can use a considerable amount of time and money, particularly when a group is being drawn together for discussion. When this situation occurs, care-giving resources are being temporarily removed from patients and the cost per person can range from $5 per hour to $30 or $40 per hour. It is an interesting and informative exercise to summarize the cost of a conference or staff meeting that lasts one hour. In these cases one must consider salaries plus fringe benefits. The fringe benefits can run 25 to 30 percent of salaries. What was accomplished by the meeting and whether or not the members fully focused on the issues that were the basis for holding the meeting in the first place must be considered. Thus, communications, whether they are written and/or oral, can be an expensive undertaking for the organization and must be accomplished in an effective manner to affect changes at a reasonable cost.

PREPAREDNESS AND EVALUATION

Perhaps one of the biggest problems for nurse-managers and society in general is the fact that communication often begins without benefit of previous thinking. So often a statement is made without thinking that feedback initially catches the manager off balance. At this stage the nurse-manager must go through a series of retransmissions to attempt to recover the situation and, following many iterations, to achieve understanding on the part of unit members. The process is unnecessary, can produce frustration, takes time, and costs money.

It is vitally important that nurse-managers devote sufficient time to preparation and forethought before communicating. The problem to be discussed should be thought through and objectives should be clearly defined. The strategy to be used following considerations of alternatives must be established. The overall acceptability of the approach and rationale must be considered. Nurse-managers should plan their communication. This approach requires some time initially but can be more effective in the end.

When the nature of the problem is such that input is necessary and desirable, managers should be most prudent not to evaluate a situation without first obtaining the requested input. If the unit members perceive that the decision has already been made or that the manager is making a premature judgement, the effectiveness of the communication will have been thwarted. The effect on future meeting input will also be grossly curtailed by unit members because the nurse-manager is not listening. In their classic article "Barriers and Gateways to Communication," Rogers and Roethlisberger (1952) have stressed the great importance of listening. In this type of situation, they suggest that each individual in the group may speak only after he or she has been able to relate the ideas and intent of the one who previously spoke. In addition, the relating of such information should be to the previous speaker's satisfaction. This approach is much more difficult than it seems initially. I suggest that this approach be used at your next meeting to experience what is actually involved in the implementation of this approach. Thus, nurse managers should not evaluate what is being said in this situation and should maintain an unbiased, uncommitted attitude until all parties involved have had full opportunity to express their points of view. This concept of listening without evaluation is a necessary condition to fostering input and enhancing the communication process.

GENERAL COMMUNICATION CONSIDERATIONS

Nurse-managers have to know where problems can occur in communications in order to anticipate them fully and to make the communication process more effective. The most obvious problem that creates a barrier to clear understanding is based on the poor use of grammar. Poorly constructed sentences and poorly used vocabulary are primary causes. The statements as constructed should be brief, clear, and to the point. Nurse-managers may often write a memorandum that is long and involved. Consequently, unit members have to ferret out the essential ideas and hope. that they have selected the correct ones. Do not leave this situation to chance; be clear and concise.

The receiver's orientation is essential in order for the nurse-manager to convey a message. The background and assumptions leading up to the issuance of the memorandum should be incorporated. Granted, such a luxury is time-consuming, but it can also be time-saving. So state your assumptions and give a brief background so that the unit members can relate to the communication and can respond from a more congruent knowledge base.

All participants in the communication process have an overriding responsibility to listen as suggested by Rogers and Roethlisberger. It is not unusual in a unit meeting to hear two members hotly debating each other on a subject that they had already agreed upon 30 minutes earlier. This type of communication activity is a waste of time for all individuals involved in the discussion.

Subject matter often has a major impact on all of the participants in a unit. The subjects could involve major staffing changes, a reorganization or merger with another hospital, for example. In such cases, nurse-managers must be careful to permit sufficient time for unit members to feel the complete effect of these possible changes. They need time to adjust psychologically to a change that may significantly affect their working conditions and responsibilities. Depending on the subject matter, it is sometimes possible over a series of meetings to prepare members of the unit psychologically about such a proposed change without having to spring the issue on them at one meeting. In other words, it is best to condition staff, if at all possible, prior to an announcement of a major change.

Thus, there are many areas that can create problems in communications, and nurse-managers must constantly strive to overcome these barriers.

THE NURSE-MANAGER AND THE GRAPEVINE

We have discussed the informal communication system of the hospital. We noted the variations of the informal system outside the formal organization and its authorized channels of communication. One of the most commonly used vehicles in the informal system is the grapevine.

The grapevine is continuously at work serving as an emotional release for unit members and can greatly assist nurse-managers in obtaining information regarding attitudes and morale of members. This implies that management must be continually attuned to the grapevine and what information it is carrying. Listening to the grapevine is an important activity if nurse-managers are to be fully informed and have a feeling for the staff and potential problems.

The grapevine can produce many rumors. Nurse-managers can use the grapevine if it is approached with care. If used correctly, it can become a very important adjunct to the formal communication channels. Many of the false rumors and misinformation being disseminated through the grapevine can be corrected by the manager. Many unit members believe greatly in the grapevine because, to a great extent, it is viewed as their communication system. For this reason, the unit members will often devote more attention to the grapevine than to the formal system. Thus, nurse-managers, in using this vehicle, can correct misinformation and perhaps secure a certain degree of attention that may not be afforded to the formal channels.

Nurse-managers have a possible role with the grapevine. Rumors that develop can be combated and the word can be passed quickly through this vehicle. Managers may want to consider the possibility of feeding and cultivating this unauthorized channel as a viable means of communicating information in a fast and informal sense. Much information can also be learned about the unit by merely listening to the grapevine.

COMMUNICATION AND EMOTION

Throughout this discussion on communication there has been a general tendency to assume that the receiver is willing to listen. The receiver has a responsibility to do his or her part in the communication process if that process is to be effective.

At this point, it is appropriate to consider that the individuals involved not be emotionally upset. For purposes of this discussion we will consider the case of oral communication. When individuals are under a high degree of stress, emotions can run high. This type of situation can result in many unintended consequences. Nurse-managers and/or unit members in a highly emotional state will tend to give directions or respond to those directions in an emotional manner rather than on a sound, rational basis. As a result, either one or both parties will make statements that they do not mean or will deliver statements in such a way that emotion will cloud the true meaning that the individual intended to convey. Both individuals will often get into such a heated discussion that neither one is listening. This situation can be observed when two individuals are shouting at each other, and both are talking at the same time. How can either one listen, when both are talking? The answer is obviously that neither one is listening. If they had been listening, they might have discovered that they had both agreed with each other two minutes ago. In this situation, the communication process is merely an opportunity for individuals to vent frustrations, and it acts as an emotional release. However, in the majority of cases, very little can be accomplished in a highly emotional state.

How can these situations be precluded in the unit? First, managers must remember that nothing will be communicated or accomplished until the emotion has been reduced. In most cases, this can be accomplished by time and distance. For example, if you enter a patient's room to find two staff members in a heated argument, one of them should be sent down the hall to take care of another patient. If you get involved in an argument of this type, separate yourself from the situation—take an elevator to the first floor and then come back. When time and distance are increased the likelihood of the highly emotional level should be measurably reduced. Many nurse-managers suggest that the discussion be continued later that day. These techniques can prove quite useful in reducing the emotion factor so that two people, as mature adults, may carry on a rational discussion and produce some effective communication.

SUMMARY

Communication is an integral part of the nurse-manager's role as a leader. Many people take communications for granted. The components of communication are a sender, receiver, message, and channel. To be an effective communicator, the sender must develop a receiver orientation before disseminating information. This approach should reduce the number of iterations necessary to clarify the message and thereby increase the effectiveness of communications.

Responsibility and accountability lie with everyone involved in the communication process. If a communication is not understood, it is the responsibility of all participants to seek clarification, or they may be held accountable for the inappropriate delivery of nursing care.

In every hospital organization there exists a formal channel of communication, which follows the formal lines of authority. Formal channels contain information authorized by management and are usually referred to as downward channels. There are also informal channels, which follow the informal organization structure. Communication in this channel is called upward channel communication since it follows up the organizational structure. The passing of information through the informal system constitutes what is known as the grapevine. The grapevine can be a faster system than the formal system. To combat this problem, management in some hospitals has incorporated a lateral information flow whereby everyone receives the information at about the same time.

Messages may either be written or oral in nature. If a record is needed, messages should be written. Oral messages have the advantage of being faster initially and providing an opportunity for immediate feedback and clarification. Written messages take longer and in some cases may be more expensive.

Communications often begin without having been thought through. Nurse-managers should plan communication by devoting enough time in preparation and forethought to ensure better acceptability and clarity. They should conduct meetings requesting input, without evaluation on a premature basis, emphasizing the need to listen if the communication process is to be effective.

Various barriers exist in communications. These barriers include content problems, poor orientation of sender, failure to listen, insufficient time for adjustment.

The grapevine, although an informal system of communication, can be most helpful to managers. Listening to the grapevine can provide insights regarding employee attitudes and feelings of staff. With reasonable care, nurse-managers can use the system to combat rumors and to disseminate information.

Effective communication cannot occur during periods of high emotion for either the sender, receiver, or both. To preclude this situation, it is necessary to put time and distance between the people so that a rational discussion may occur and effective communication can become a reality.

BIBLIOGRAPHY

Alter, Steven L. "How Effective Managers Use Information Systems." *Harvard Business Review*, vol. 54, no. 6 (November–December 1976): 97–104.

Douglass, Laura Mae, and Bevis, Em Olivia. *Nursing Leadership in Action*, 2nd ed. St. Louis: C. V. Mosby, 1974.

Koontz, Harold, and O'Donnell, Cyril. *Management: A Systems and Contingency Analysis of Managerial Functions*, 6th ed. New York: McGraw-Hill, 1976.

Lewis, G. K. "Communication, A Factor in Meeting Emotional Crises." *Nursing Outlook* 13 (1965): 36–39.

Rogers, Carl R., and Roethlisberger, F. J. "Barriers and Gateways to Communications." *Harvard Business Review*, vol. 30, no. 4 (July-August 1952): 46–52.

Ruesch, J., and Bateson, G. *Communication: The Social Matrix of Psychiatry*. New York: Norton, 1968.

Strausmann, Paul A. "Managing the Costs of Information." *Harvard Business Review*, vol. 54, no. 5 (September–October 1976): 133–142.

Tannenbaum, Robert.; Weschler, I. R., and Massarik, Fred. *Leadership and Organization: A Behavioral Approach*. New York: McGraw-Hill, 1961.

Chapter 18

Effective Group
Dynamics in Nursing

"At the present time, nursing is performed by a group of nurses who are striving to help the client achieve his health-care goals" (Yura, Ozimek & Walsh, 1976, p. 116). The practice of nursing is essentially group and interpersonally oriented. In the last chapter we discussed the role of communication from an interpersonal basis. Now we shall examine the practice of nursing from the group orientation. Nurse managers are constantly working with groups—with colleagues on the unit or with other health-care providers or patients. Nurse-managers must be able to operate effectively within the various structures of nursing care—case, functional, team method, and primary-care methods. In all delivery systems, groups are an integral part of each system. For our purposes, we will define a group as two or more individuals who interact and are interdependent and who work together toward a common objective.

The early writings in management that viewed the group as an important consideration for management were published in the mid-1920s to the late 1930s (Follett, 1924; Mayo, 1933; Barnard, 1938). During that period of time the study of groups and group dynamics became a separate field of research and study under the guidance and direction of Kurt Lewin. Since then many universities have developed centers to study the phenomena of group dynamics.

Groups are formed for various purposes. Some groups exist for management-identified, specific reasons and become part of the formal organization. Other groups form voluntarily and constitute the informal structure of organizations. The formal group may be assigned certain managerial-type functions with decision-making authority, whereas others are permitted to deliberate problems and make recommendations to management. Other formal groups are for information exchange. Thus, formal groups do have various levels of authority and responsibility within the organizational structure. Informal groups have no formal delegated authority but may have significant influence and power depending on the composition of the group and the particular issue under consideration at that time.

ADVANTAGES OF GROUPS

There are many advantages to the use of groups in nursing, which explains their extensive use in nursing units and departments. The most obvious reason for groups is the collective thought process that occurs through consideration of problems and the effective exercising of sound judgement. We have all experienced the group process that has operated well by bringing together individuals with diverse experience and education. As a result of this process, more ideas and opinions are generated; the group tends to examine the problem at greater length; and the combined effect provides a judgement level which exceeds that attainable by a single individual working alone. This point was well stated by Jay (1971, p. 19), "Although an idea can originate in one person's mind, it can be greatly improved if six or seven people question and add to it, elaborate on and refine it."

The group process can act as a vehicle to stimulate individuals by permitting a greater degree of involvement in organizational activities that would not have been possible without the group. Through this involvement aspect of group processes, individuals can become motivated and committed to the implementation phase of projects. In essence, the individuals who were involved in the group would like to see their ideas and suggestions come to fruition. Generally, they will work hard to make sure that the ideas become a reality through action.

In other situations groups can greatly assist management in the coordination of internal plans and programs. For example, a benevolent-autocrat-type manager may form a group to assist management in the implementation and coordination of those plans when plans have been almost exclusively developed by management. Managers usually take this step because they realize the need for others to be involved in order to carry out the plan as conceived. This form of partial involvement is somewhat helpful in motivating individuals, but it does not seem to have as great a motivational impact as involving individuals early on—at the idea stage of development. Certainly, however, even some involvement is better than none. Involvement provides definite evidence to unit members that their opinions are valued by management.

The use of groups permits the individuals in the group to develop a degree of loyalty toward each other as well as a sense of responsibility for the group decisions. Through this group process an esprit de corps is developed, and the group establishes a feeling of work as a team with a resulting increase in group cohesiveness. The extent of cohesiveness generally depends on the amount of involvement and the degree to which the group activities can assist the individual in meeting individual needs. As more individual needs can be met, the more cohesive the group, the greater the motivational level to accomplish the objectives of the group.

Nurse-managers can learn much about individuals by observing their behavior in groups. Anyone who has worked with groups knows that, in the vast majority of cases, the group vehicle usually provides a forum for leadership to emerge. The individual who merely verbally dominates the group will not necessarily emerge as a leader. Rather, the individual who is listened to by the other members is a leader. The individual who, through proper use of human relations skills, can assist the group in reaching compromises without great sacrifice to either side is a leader. Thus, the group process permits nurse-managers with a laboratorylike setting to watch for the development of leaders in the unit, and helps in determining those individuals who have power through respect of their colleagues.

Finally, groups are very useful management tools for the exchange of information. With all parties involved present, managers can convey and receive information so that all unit members are informed of a situation simultaneously. Feedback and clarification for all members can occur within a reasonably short period of time without having to provide the same explanation on numerous occasions. Thus, a certain degree of efficiency in communication can be secured, while the loss of status from being the last individual to get the information can be prevented.

DISADVANTAGES OF GROUPS

Perhaps one of the greatest disadvantages to the use of groups is the splitting of responsibility, which leads to reduced concern by individuals for problems being deliberated or decisions being made. The more traditionally-oriented nurse-managers believe this situation to be a definite problem because only individuals, not groups, bear the burden of responsibility. On the other hand, a more behaviorally oriented nurse-manager would not necessarily view the acceptance of responsibility by a group as a problem. These two opposing viewpoints are certainly debatable. As a nurse-manager how do you feel about this question? Can an individual participating as a member of a group feel as responsible for recommendations or decisions, as the person who will be held solely responsible for the results of such recommendations or decisions?

In terms of time and money the cost of groups can be considerable. This situation can be exacerbated when the group tends to be ineffective through overdeliveration of problems. In addition, some group recommendations or decisions may be impractical in terms of implementation. Some individuals tend to take up considerable time in group sessions because they merely want to talk. This situation wastes everyone's time, including the speaker, although there may be some therapeutic side effects for the speaker.

In group processes individual members tend to argue; consequently, many members may withhold their own personal views to preclude conflict which can result in an uncomfortable situation. This kind of stifling effect, which is generally self-imposed, can result in the group accepting a less forceful position than might have been determined by an individual nurse-manager. It is not unusual to see groups take positions, after much deliberation, that tend to be quite weak and conservative. This implies that most changes proposed by groups in general will not have a tremendous impact on the status quo. Thus, the deliberative/interactive process of groups can foster argument while demonstrating successive conformity and weakness of results.

Groups can be used incorrectly by nurse-managers to gain additional power. If nurse managers lead groups without much opportunity for input, and enforce their own views, the groups will merely become fronts for nurse-managers. This type of ploy indicates that the results were a collective group decision. Individuals are merely going through an exercise to meet the power needs of their nurse-manager. Those individuals who were not part of the group will be misled by the fact that the conclusion was a direct result of active group deliberation. This problem is made worse when one considers the fact that the results of group decisions usually have a higher degree of acceptance by others because more people are involved in a group decision. Thus, it is most important that nurse-managers use groups in an appropriate manner and permit good active involvement by group members.

CONSIDERATIONS FOR EFFECTIVE GROUPS

In working with groups nurse-managers must be aware of the vital role of the chairperson. To a great extent, the chairperson will determine the overall success of the group. Since nurse-managers will fill the role of chairperson on many occasions, learning to perform effectively in this position is essential. The chairperson must plan the meetings of groups, not merely let them happen. The amount of preparation will vary depending on the purpose of the meeting. Different applications for meetings and conferences will be discussed later in this chapter. The chairperson must perform a balancing act during a meeting to make sure that as many individuals as possible participate within given time constraints. In some cases the discussion may become quite one-sided on a situation. At this point, it is incumbent on the chairperson to play the other side, by acting as a devil's advocate. The group discussion should be kept to the subject at hand to maintain relevancy and progress toward meeting objectives. Following group discussions, the chairperson has the responsibility to provide the group with a summation of the discussion in an unbiased manner. During the summation phase, the chairperson must effectively integrate the ideas presented and, if possible, provide direction for the finalization of the group's deliberations. Thus, the role of the chairperson cannot be overemphasized because of its great importance.

In many nursing staff situations involving the use of groups, the number of group members may be predetermined (i.e., number of staff for a conference). In situations in which the number of participants can be established by the chairperson, it is suggested that the group not be too large. Certainly, enough individuals should be included so that all possible differing points of view may be represented. At the same time, it must be remembered that the more people involved, the less the involvement in discussion is possible by each member. Individuals can get lost in large groups and feel that their viewpoint would not be that important. In addition, they feel that other members of the group will probably express the views they would have proposed. Thus, with large groups a dilution of individually-felt responsibility can occur. In order to secure a good balance of representation while providing an opportunity for involvement, it is necessary that the group not be too large. It has been suggested that a group size of five members is ideal for sufficient representation (Filley, 1970; Porter, 1963). Another researcher has recommended that groups have six to ten members (Bonner, 1959). Research has given us a variety of group sizes, although one optimal size has not been universally obtained. Sound judgement using the principles provided and the conditions of the situation will assist nurse-managers greatly in making an appropriate decision about the size of the group.

The nature and purpose of the group should be clearly defined. The role and responsibility must be aligned with the authority provided to the group. The purpose can be to give input to the nurse manager. On the other hand, detailed recommendations may be explicitly set forth. In addition, the group could have the direct charge of making a decision relevant to a pertinent pressing issue. Thus, nurse-managers must ascertain and specifically state the purpose, role, responsibility, and authority of the group and ensure that the factors are understood by all members of the group.

Finally, nurse-managers must exercise prudence in the use of groups. Previously, we stressed the need for involvement in the decision-making process of individuals on the unit and in the department. This facet of organizational life is certainly true; however, it is necessary to realize that leadership is primarily a quality of the individual. With this concept in mind, there are many situations and decisions that can be handled quite adequately by managers without calling a group together. In some cases, little, if any, consultation might be necessary. In other cases, input may be desirable but can be handled perhaps more effectively on a disaggregated basis. The nurse-manager would meet individually with a few members of the unit to obtain their viewpoints and consultation without bringing a whole group together. Therefore, it is necessary that forethought be given as to whether a group is really needed for the proper handling of the issue under consideration. Time and experience will greatly help in making sound judgements in these areas. In general, decisions that can be properly made by nurse-managers should be made by them.

NURSING CONFERENCES

Many organizations have various types of groups that meet for many reasons. For nurse-managers, the most common type of group is the formally organized conference.

These conferences take on many forms depending on the needs of the situation. Although these conferences are formally organized, the meetings themselves tend to be conducted in an informal way. The conferences are usually relatively short—from 20 to 30 minutes. The members of the unit and nurse-managers are placed under a great many demands every day; therefore, their time is precious, and the meeting, though informal, should be conducted in an efficient manner. It should keep to the subjects at hand, and comments should be brief and to the point. It is important in preparing assignments of personnel, that managers provide sufficient staffing for patient care during the period of the conference. This planning will permit those members attending the conference to devote their full attention to the meeting. If this staffing coverage does not occur, the unit members will have difficulty becoming effectively involved in the group process.

At the beginning of each shift nurse-managers will hold a conference to plan the unit operations for that shift. Nurse-managers will take the functions to be performed and make staffing assignments including areas of responsibility based on current patient load and acuity. Other information is disseminated at that time, which should assist staff in carrying out patient-care responsibilities. A portion of these meetings can be planned by nurse-managers based on the report of the conference of the previous shift. In addition, physician orders, including tests, should be incorporated into the planning process. As a capstone to the planning, nurse-managers should validate all relevant information about patients' conditions and progress by conducting their own assessment of all patients on the unit through the visitation. Once this information has been obtained and validated, and nurse-manager assessment completed, the initial planning has been completed. Due to the dynamic nature of the nursing environment, a portion of the meeting cannot be planned or anticipated. Consequently, there must be on-site adjustments during the conference to meet unanticipated and unplanned factors in the environment. The factors can include scheduled staff who do not appear or emergency admissions that are referred to the unit. Adjustments in assignments and responsibilities must be made to ensure appropriate patient coverage and the best use of staffing resources.

It is important that reasons and rationale be given to staff members for the decisions being made even though the time for these meetings is quite short. The rationale given can often increase understanding and commitment in carrying out the directives of management. In addition, nurse-managers should demonstrate sensitivity toward the staff members in consideration of their longevity on the unit and of their general understanding of organizational policies and procedures, including unit protocol. In the case of relatively new personnel on the unit, greater detailed explanations are necessary to achieve the same level of understanding as that of more experienced personnel. Nurse-managers handle this problem either through the conference itself or by having a brief discussion after the conference to clear up certain situations with any individuals who need more explanation.

Nurse-managers are also actively involved in conferences relating to specific cases on the unit, which provides an effective teaching/learning situation for staff members and can result in recommendations to enhance the quality of nursing care delivered to patients. In these situations, nurse-managers and staff collectively use all the nursing process to assess the patient's condition, to identify patient problems, develop nursing-care plans with elaborated rationale, provide mechanisms for intervention and

evaluation. This type of experience for staff members can be quite beneficial. The experience is helpful in enhancing the ability of staff to identify
problems and solve them through the use of nursing principles. As chairperson of the case conference, nurse-managers should present the
background of the situation and then let unit members actively work
through the nursing process. Using a theoretical framework to think
through the case provides an excellent environment for learning by active
involvement. For others, the active involvement will reinforce previous
knowledge and greatly increase recall in future cases.

The case conference can often act as a spark to motivate unit members to learn more about a certain disease and treatment. In addition, it
may even result in a request for an in-depth presentation of a topic. Thus,
the case conference can be the start of foundation for future content
conferences, which can be planned at a convenient time for staff attendance. The amount of interest demonstrated by nurse-managers will
greatly help to inspire staff members to attend the content conferences
and will foster a teaching/learning environment. Nurse-managers should
promote these sessions and show their commitment by having them
scheduled on a regular basis. These conference presentations assist staff
in developing a wider and more in-depth knowledge from which they can
draw and improve the quality of care delivered. There is usually a certain
amount of preparation necessary to make content conferences effective.
Unit members will generally know when a presenter has not done their
"homework." Well-prepared presentations will act to motivate unit
members to give better care and assure future attendance at content conferences. The nurse manager's role is similar to a case conference with
active involvement from unit members. The duration of the conference,
depending on subject matter, can run from 45 minutes to an hour.

At the conclusion of a shift, nurse-managers will convene staff members for report. The report conference acts as a forum for the exchange of
information regarding events that occurred during the shift. This conference is a period of information-sharing with other members of the unit.
The report includes progress reports of care to patients in consideration of
patient-care objectives, observations and clinical objective data, and an
opportunity to iterate nursing-care plans to reflect changing patient conditions. As mentioned previously, the "report" is one of the principal input
devices for conducting the conference at the beginning of the next shift.
Thus, the report conference is vital to ensuring the effectiveness of the
next shift's opening conference through the change-of-shift report. The
principal role of the nurse-manager in the report conference is to listen
and provide guidance on specifics that may not have been included in the
initial report. This probing-type of questioning is used to clarify issues and
in some cases is designed as an educational device for other unit mem-

bers. Certainly, the time period of the report is short and each member has much information to present. Therefore, it is strongly suggested that nurse-managers assist members by expressing certain expectations before the actual reporting. If nurse-managers state their expectations early on, they will save time and have a more effective report conference.

The final conference that we will consider is the problem-solving conference. These conferences are called by nurse-managers to address problems that have developed in the working environment. The problems presented can relate to dynamics of the group, specific interpersonal problems, procedures, policies, product or equipment problems on the unit. It is most important the nurse-managers fully delineate the role and authority being assigned as part of the statement of the problem. Such a statement of expectations, including operational parameters, should facilitate the functioning of the group. Nurse-managers should not approach the apparent problem with many preconceived notions. As the discussion begins to evolve, it is not unusual to find that the apparent problem may not, in fact, be the real problem. In other cases, the apparent problem may be the real problem, but through the discussion, many tangential and related problems may come to light. Through an active and open interchange of ideas and observations, much can be learned about feelings and attitudes as well as discovering how the unit actually operates from the unit members' perspective. In many cases during the discussion, nurse-managers can effectively, assist the members in articulating problems through proper questioning without making evaluations or conclusions. Managers should make sure that all individuals in the group become involved in this discussion. This may require some proving and drawing of information from individuals to secure maximal participation from all concerned. It is important that all members carry the load of responsibility and that the discussion not be dominated by a few members. Nurse-managers must develop certain leadership skills to conduct problem-solving conferences effectively. These skills include such techniques as drawing information from "quiet" members, giving a question to an individual who has not stated a position on that issue (consultative opinion from third party), asking general questions to the whole group without specifically addressing it to any particular individual, and restating a question back to the originator in a question by asking his or her opinion. All of these techniques can be used in most problem-solving conferences.

Once the problem(s) has been identified and alternatives considered, groups should collectively attempt to reach a consensus. When the consensus has been obtained, nurse-managers should indicate what specific steps will be taken to consider further or to implement the solution developed by the group. This conclusion of a group meeting is necessary to establish the finality element of the conference. This element provides feedback to the members that their time and effort were for a purpose, while providing a feeling of self-worth to the individuals involved in the conference.

SUMMARY

Nursing practice is group and interpersonally oriented. Groups are an integral part of all health-care delivery systems. Some groups are formal in nature and exist for identified management purposes; other groups are informal and are a natural consequence of the informal organization. Formal groups are assigned authority and responsibility by management.

Nursing uses many groups because of the apparent advantages. Collective thought enhances judgement for decision making. Involvement in the group stimulates and motivates individuals, assists in coordination, increases cohesiveness among unit members, facilitates understanding of individual member behavior, helps in leader identification, and finally enhances the exchange of information.

There are certain disadvantages to the use of groups in nursing which include splitting of responsibility; time cost; conformity of views and weakness of recommendations and decisions; and incorrect use of power.

For groups to be effective the following considerations are necessary. First, the role of the chairperson is vital to the success of the group. Second, the size of the group should be kept relatively small, if at all possible. Third, the nature and purpose of the group must be clear and understood by all participants. Fourth, groups should not be used to replace the nurse-manager's decision-making role. Decisions that can be properly made by nurse-managers should be made by them.

In the practical applications in the nursing unit of groups, the conference is the prevailing form. Conferences used in the unit include conferences at the beginning of each shift (to make staffing assignments and assign responsibility), case conferences (to review specific patient cases that provide a teaching/learning situation for staff members and many times enhance the quality of care delivered), content conferences (presentation of specific content matter to increase knowledge and understanding of staff), report conferences (forum for exchange of information pertaining to events that occurred during the shift), and the problem-solving conference (to explore problems and to develop solutions relating to problems in group dynamics, interpersonal problems, procedures, policies, product or equipment problems).

In almost all conferences the duration of the meeting is short, informal, and nurse-managers must plan the conduct of the conference in order for them to be meaningful and effective.

BIBLIOGRAPHY

Barnard, Chester I. *The Functions of the Executive*. Cambridge, Mass: Harvard University Press, 1938.

Bonner, H. *Group Dynamics*. New York: The Ronald Press, 1959.

Cartwright, D., and Zander, A., eds. *Group Dynamics: Research and Theory*, 3rd ed. New York: Harper & Row, 1968.

Follett, Mar Parker. *Creative Experience*. New York: Longmans, Green, 1924.

Filley, A. C. "Committee Management: Guidelines from Social Science Research". *California Management Review*, vol. 13, no. 1 (Fall 1970): 13–21.

Jay, Antone. *Corporation Man*. New York: Random House, 1971.

Mayo, Elton. *The Human Problems of an Industrial Civilization*. Cambridge, Mass.: Harvard University Press, 1933.

Porter, D. E. "Information Distribution and Group Size." *Industrial Management Review*, vol. 4, no. 2 (Spring 1963): 1–17.

Yura, Helen; Ozimek, Dorothy; and Walsh, Mary B. *Nursing Leadership: Theory and Process*. New York: Appleton-Century-Crofts, 1976.

Zander, A. *Motives and Goals in Groups*. New York: Academic Press, 1971.

Part Five

Controlling in Nursing

Part Five is designed to provide information and concepts relating to the last managerial function to be considered—controlling. The formal development of control systems must include the nature and process of controls as well as some formal nursing control system considerations (Section A). The behavioral influences on such formal control systems can be substantial and are considered from the standpoint of nurse interface with controls, change theory and change agents, and the organization of the informal organization (Section B).

Chapter 19 reviews the nature and process of general control systems. The process of control includes a measurable standard, comparison mechanism, and effectuating systemic changes to correct deviations from standards. In addition, control system considerations are discussed at length.

Chapter 20 addresses formal nursing control systems. Areas of discussion include structure-process-outcome triad, nursing audit as a management tool, professional standards review organizations, nursing quality control systems, and functional system/quality interface.

Chapter 21 examines the interface of the nurse with the control system. The symptoms of interface control problems are discussed including early and later stage indicators as well as generalized symptoms. An analysis of crisis management is covered as well as a prognosis for the nurse manager. The final section considers nurse-managers' attitudes toward staff with the conclusion that staff behavior is, to a great degree, dependent on the tone set by management.

Chapter 22 discusses change theory and change agents in nursing. Topic areas include the need for change, resistance to change, management of change, management of conflict, and organization development.

In the final chapter (23), the organization of the informal organization is addressed. The dissatisfaction of staff evolves into a more formal structure with the development of labor unions in the hospital setting. The impact of the union movement since the removal of exemption for hospitals under the Taft-Hartley Act is considered at length.

Formal Controlling

Chapter 19

Nature and Process of Control Systems

Nurse-managers have not generally been exposed to the concept of managerial control. The most recent publications on nursing management and leadership appear to be devoid of this vital management function. Perhaps the closest reference to control has been expressed through discussions relating to the need for coordination (Eckelberry, 1971, Chapter 10). As we shall see later, coordination is a part of the control function. Generally, the control function monitors the system and through efforts of the nurse manager, facilitates the integration of activities on the unit. Control is the last of the management functions to be considered.

Control is a closely related function to planning for nurse-managers. The planning function provides the basis upon which the control function is predicated. Similarly, through its feedback mechanism the control process can provide input from the output function to establish the need to modify and adjust organizational plans.

NATURE OF CONTROL

Once plans are developed, organizing has occurred, directing has been established, nurse-managers must know how everything is going. The control function of management addresses this problem. Control represents that aspect of the total management process which assists the nurse-manager in maintaining unit and department activity within the bounds of expectations. Control, then, is principally focused on ensuring that plans are being met as originally conceived.

Coordination, as a subpart of control, is directed toward the proper orchestration of multiple unit activities within a specific time frame. Proper coordination occurs when management has established the sequencing of activities with specified target times. The three management functions of planning, organizing, and directing constitute the basis for the orchestration of activities. Coordination tells the nurse-manager that certain activities are being performed in an intended sequence and on a timely basis. In essence, coordination is ensuring that the management process is operating in an orderly and appropriate fashion.

The remaining portion of the control function is examining the outcome of the process to determine if expectations are being met. This aspect of control incorporates the testing and comparison of results with planned objectives. Thus, the final analysis is the results-determination phase of the control function.

To ensure that the nurse-manager has effective control of operations, both coordination (process) and outcome (results) must be an integral part of this function. In order for nurse-managers to develop controls, certain preconditions must exist. The controls as conceived must be predicated on the existence of plans. Without proper planning how can nurse-managers establish the current status of the system? They must be able to measure progress against benchmarks, to ascertain that there are deviations from expectations or to determine that objectives are being met. Likewise, the greater the detailed planning that has been performed, the better the control mechanisms. Thus, planning plays a key role in the design of management control systems.

In a similar manner the organizing process is important to the development of proper control systems. Organizing should precede work on control function aspects of organizations. The more thought is devoted to functions and functionalization, the more logical will be the assignment of roles. The more definitive the roles, the more specific the assignment of responsibility and authority. Thus, the clearer, the more definitive and integrated the organizing process and resulting structure, the better the elaboration and effectiveness of control systems. With properly developed plans and organizational structure, nurse-managers can actively pursue the design and development of control systems.

Organizations through their control function exhibit homeostasis-type and dynamic equilibrium-type properties. We know from study of the living process of human beings that homeostasis exists. Organisms of human beings have mechanisms of control that tend to be self-regulating and make necessary systemic corrections to maintain a dynamic equilibrium through the life of a human being. Organizations have similar properties but do not demonstrate the exactness of human organisms because of the social nature of organizations. Certainly, organizations through policies and procedures have a suggested normal state of affairs for situations. Variations from those policies and procedures usually result in some within-organizational correction to return to the preferred state. In the majority of cases, functioning in the organization is conducted within the accepted boundaries and thereby maintains a stability of actions over time. Thus, there exists a tendency toward a steady state, in its simplest form, which is homeostatic in nature, to maintain the organizational system. In addition, the organization is continuously exposed to stimuli from both within and outside the organization. The impact of these stimuli are such as to generally preclude the return of the organization to its original state of equilibrium (Lewin, 1947). From the standpoint of system theory, we have described a dynamic homeostasis because the state of equilibrium is being maintained through a process of adjustment over time. We observe this condition in nursing units as the social system and its constituent subsystems have their own complexity of motivational forces moving toward new equilibrium levels on a continuous basis. Nursing organizations are changing and adjusting over time and should be considered as being in a state of dynamic equilibrium.

Another aspect of establishing control systems is the cybernetic concept. Wiener (1948, 1954) has observed that communication and control exist in many systems: physical, biological, and social. In his work he demonstrated that systems have control features through information feedback that identify deviations from expectations and incorporate corrective procedures. Thus, the system will exert effort (energy) to feedback information for corrective purposes. Management control, then, is that part of the total management system which monitors performance and feeds back information that is used to modify and adjust plans, organizational structure, and directing functions.

PROCESS OF CONTROL

Management control systems consist of a series of elements that operate through a process. The elements of the control process are: (1) a measurable standard or characteristic, (2) a comparison mechanism for comparing results to standards and performing an evaluation of established differentials, and (3) effecting systemic changes to correct deviations from standards. This process is used in all organizational settings regardless of complexity or activity level.

Nurse-managers function in a unit setting that was described as in a state of dynamic equilibrium. As such, portions of their daily work consist of supervising and observing the performance of unit members caring for patients. Since the complexity of the operating environment is so great, it is not possible to observe all of the activity occurring on the unit. Hence, a good portion of patient care is conducted by staff without the benefit of nurse-manager direct supervision or guidance. Therefore, it is necessary to establish standards as measures to provide criteria for performance of staff on the unit. The standards as developed provide a basis on which to measure progress and performance. If at all possible, the standards should be stated in objective, verifiable terms, preferably quantitatively-oriented, although some may have to be qualitative in nature. Standards that are couched in terms of objectives and results give the nurse-manager the best basis for control purposes. Generally, standards of performance based on objectives will fall into the following categories: (1) quality of nursing care, (2) quantity of nursing care, and (3) timeliness of performance. To a great extent many experts in quality of nursing care believe, and rightly so, that timeliness is an integral part of the quality of care delivered. The third category was given to highlight the great importance of timing to performance. Depending on the criticalness of a patient's condition, timeliness can be of extreme importance.

The next step in the process of control is the comparative function of measuring the actual results obtained to the established standards. At this point, the nurse-manager is receiving feedback information from the unit indicating that deviations have occurred. An evaluation should be performed to ascertain the scope and magnitude of the deviation. Next, an estimate is made of the potential impact on the system. The information for evaluation emanates from control points. As part of the management process these points constitute the time and place where formal feedback occurs to assist the nurse-manager. Obviously, not all points in the process are important to the overall effective operation of the unit. For this reason, prudent nurse-managers will purposely design and select points that are strategic to the proper functioning of the unit. The selection of strategic control points should take into consideration that the activities are primary to the success of the unit. The activities being covered should be balanced, including varied functions, and they should be comprehensive in nature, so that minor activities do not activate feedback information that is not material to overall operations. The timing of the initiation of the feedback must be sufficiently early in the process so that adequate time remains to effect systemic changes. Thus, the time for feedback should be established well in advance of the target date for completion of the objective. The earlier in the system that significant feedback can be generated, the greater the managerial opportunity to make systemic corrections that will be meaningful. As Koontz and O'Donnell (1976, p.646) state, "Intelligent and alert managers have recognized that the only problems they can solve are those they can see . . . in the case of management control . . . they can exercise it effectively only if they can see deviations coming in time to do something about them." Koontz and O'Donnell suggest that managers should use a feedforward (rather than feedback) approach to control because most "feedback is not much more than a postmortem, and no one has found a way to change the past" (Koontz & O'Donnell, 1976, p.646). In feedforward control, the manager is constantly monitoring the inputs of the process to ascertain deviations. A rather elaborate set of requirements for feedforward control is recommended. For our purposes it is strongly suggested that meaningful feedback be established through strategic control points early enough in the process to institute some meaningful and measurable change.

The final step in the control process is effecting change to correct deviations from standards. A good portion of the feedback received by the nurse-manager indicates that objectives are being met on schedule. Here we are interested in the situations in which deviations from expectations have occurred and require some type of managerial corrective action. Once the deviation has been identified, the nurse-manager should ascertain what courses of action are appropriate to alleviate and correct the situation. Certainly, the unit that has completed the planning function and organizing phase of management well, will be able to pinpoint the reason for the deviation and to correct it more easily. Depending on the situation, management may want to redefine its objectives and plans because they may not be appropriate for that time and place. Functions should also be analyzed again for appropriateness. Perhaps reexamination of assignments of roles and responsibilities may be needed. Unit members may need additional training and education. They may not be performing up to expectation, and termination of those members may be an appropriate managerial action. On the other hand, perhaps the unit members did not understand their roles and responsibilities because they had not been properly communicated by nurse-managers. A further detailed explanation of roles and responsibilities may be required. Thus, many possible managerial actions can be taken. The actions are dependent on the needs of the situation as best identified by the nurse manager.

CONTROL SYSTEM CONSIDERATIONS

When the nurse-manager is working on the design and development of control systems there are many considerations that justify time and effort. First, the procedures as conceived in the planning phase should be simple and understandable. If the procedures are complex, the probability of successful implementation is substantially reduced. The number of procedures should be kept to a minimum. In some units the number of procedures has become so great that staff feel overwhelmed and tend to ignore them. Therefore, the number of procedures should be staff manageable. The procedures should also be clear and concise so that management and staff can understand them and be able to perform effectively within those guidelines. It is important that these aspects be considered, because if the procedures are not implemented, nurse-managers have lost an essential element of control.

Second, the procedures used for control should be flexible. The process and outcome measures must permit adjustment for changing conditions. With the great number of changes occurring in health-care delivery, and in particular in nursing-care delivery, the procedures governing unit operations may become absolute in a relatively short period of time. For this reason, nurse-managers must view procedures in a dynamic sense so that possible revisions are considered on a continuous basis.

Third, functions are redefined and roles of staff are changed from time to time. When roles are redesigned and responsibilities are reassigned, it is important then that unit procedures be reviewed to make sure that they remain relevant. It is important to view the procedures used in the unit as a system. Changes in one procedure may very well interface with other procedures and produce changes in other procedures. Thus, the procedures which are principally administrative and in some cases clinical should be aligned with the formal structure of the unit. Remember there should be a priority of authority and responsibility. As implementation mechanisms, procedures also must conform to the authority delegated and responsibility assigned to staff members.

Fourth, nurse-managers have a responsibility carefully to examine procedures from a total-systems point of view. In many cases, the procedures as conceived partially duplicate other procedures. Procedures can also overlap other procedures and can conflict. A periodic review of all procedures is necessary to ensure that these conditions do not exist. Nurse-managers who perform a comprehensive review of procedures will find that the resulting revised procedures are simpler in nature and tend to reduce confusion in their implementation. These reviews are best performed quarterly to ensure timeliness and appropriateness of procedures.

Fifth, the concept of control used will depend to a great extent on the managerial leadership style and the amount of staff involvement in the planning and control function design. As you will recall, McGregor (1960) conceived two theories of human motivation—Theory X and Theory Y. Under Theory X, individuals had to be coerced and controlled. With Theory Y, individuals possessed an intrinsic interest in their work. As a result, individuals tended to be self-motivated and self-directed.

Employees also sought out responsibility and demonstrated self-control. If the concept of self-control can be fostered by nurse-managers through a Theory-Y orientation, then the direct supervisory role of nurse-managers can be substantially reduced. The individual staff members will exhibit self-control and will call nurse-managers attention to potential problems before they materialize. This form of early notification will enhance management effectiveness since managers will be able to take appropriate corrective action to affect change.

Nurse-managers can only hope to realize this type of staff behavior, if the leadership style used involves staff in the development of plans and control systems. Staff involvement in these procedures is important to securing the commitment and motivation to improve the system through elements of self-control. Thus, nurse-managers who approach the staff with a democratic leadership style coupled with a Theory Y orientation will help establish greater control of unit operations through the staff members motivated to control their own performance.

Sixth, the final consideration in developing control systems is the informal organizational structure. As previously mentioned, control systems should be aligned with the formal structure of authority and responsibility. In a similar manner, to the extent that the informal structure differs from the formal, nurse-managers should consider these aspects in designing control systems. Recall that the system of operation of the unit does not strictly follow the formal organizational structure, but, rather, it is an integration of both the formal and informal structures. For that reason, nurse-managers should include their knowledge of the informal structure in designing control systems in the unit and department.

SUMMARY

Control is one of the four basic management functions. The control function monitors the operation of the system primarily through nurse-managers who act as facilitators to integrate unit activities. Basically, control focuses on whether plans are being met.

Coordination concerns the proper orchestration of many activities within certain time frames. As part of the control function, coordination is the process that ties together the functions of planning, organizing, and directing.

The outcome portion of control includes the testing and comparison of results with planned objectives. Congruency of results with objectives indicates conformity with expectations. Lack of conformity implies a need for managerial action to correct the system.

The planning function is closely linked to control activities. Planning provides the operational basis for the existence of control procedures. Organizing and directing functions also play an important role in control.

Organizations exhibit homeostasis-type and dynamic equilibrium-type behavior. Through their change and adjustment behavior over time, nursing organizations are considered to be in a state of dynamic equilibrium.

Control systems include a process consisting of elements—a standard, comparative mechanism and corrective action by management. Standards of performance based on objectives include quality and quantity of nursing care as well as the timeliness of performance.

The concepts of feedback and feedforward techniques provide an opportunity to undertake corrective action. The earlier in the system that information can be generated, the greater is the managerial opportunity to make systemic corrections that will be meaningful. Management corrective actions may take a variety of forms from redesigning plans and organizational structures to the termination of staff members.

There are many considerations in developing control systems: procedures should be simple and understandable; procedures should be flexible in design; procedures must follow authority and responsibility lines; total system review is necessary on a periodic basis; managerial leadership style and involvement affect the amount of self-control; and informal aspects of organizations influence control design considerations.

BIBLIOGRAPHY

Ackoff, Russell L. *A Concept of Corporate Planning*. New York: Wiley-Interscience, 1970.

Anthony, R. N. *Planning and Control Systems: A Framework for Analysis*. Cambridge, Mass. Division of Research, Harvard Business School, 1965.

Durbin, Richard L., and Springall, W. H. *Organization and Administration of Health Care: Theory, Practice, Environment*. St. Louis: C. V. Mosby, 1969.

Drucker, P. F. *Management: Tasks, Responsibilities, and Practices*. New York: Harper & Row, 1973.

Eckelberry, Grace K. *Administration of Comprehensive Nursing Care*. New York: Appleton-Century-Crofts, 1971.

Kast, F. E., and Rosenzweig, James E. *Organization and Management: A Systems Approach*. New York: McGraw-Hill, 1970.

Koontz, H., and Bradspies, R. W. "Managing through Feedforward Control." *Business Horizons,* vol. 15, no. 3 (June 1972): 25–36.

———— and O'Donnell, C. *Management: A Systems and Contingency Analysis of Managerial Functions,* 6th ed. New York: McGraw-Hill, 1976.

Lewin, K. "Frontiers in Group Dynamics." *Human Relations* 1 (1947): 5–41.

McGregor, Douglas. *The Human Side of Enterprise*. New York: McGraw-Hill, 1960.

Schulz, Rockwell, and Johnson, Alton C. *Management of Hospitals*. New York: McGraw-Hill, 1976.

Slee, V. N. "How to Know If You Have Quality Control." *Hospital Progress,*
    vol. 53, no. 1 (1972). 38–43.
Wiener, Norbert. *Cybernetics: Control and Communication in the Animal and
    the Machine.* New York:, 1948.
_____. *The Human Use of Human Beings,* rev. ed. Boston: Houghton Mifflin,
    1954.

Chapter 20

Formal Nursing Control Systems

Previously we considered the general nature and process of control systems. Now we will examine formal nursing control systems. As part of the total control function, control processes constitute an integral portion of our primary consideration. The results of nursing care as compared to projected outcome criteria comprise the remaining portion of the control function. Basically, the approach used here will relate to the performance of groups of nurses and nursing personnel. However, we cannot forget the role of individual responsibility and accountability. An earlier chapter related individual performance to effective performance appraisal in nursing. Here the focus will address the control of nursing-care delivery by groups of nurses to ensure that optimal nursing-care delivery may become a reality.

STRUCTURE-PROCESS-OUTCOME TRIAD

Earlier we noted that management control systems consisted of a series of elements that operated through a process, in our case, the nursing process. Likewise, nursing outcome criteria (Berg, 1974; Lewis, 1974; Zimmer, 1974) and structure should be examined to obtain more of the total picture of the nursing care delivered. In other words, can quality nursing care be delivered if expected outcomes cannot be achieved? Certainly, from the outset it is fully recognized that not all patient-care factors are controllable. On the other hand, this reason alone cannot be used in all cases for unanticipated consequences. Much research has been conducted to ascertain measures of the quality of nursing care. Quality is the central goal of nursing units.

Donabedian (1969, pp. 2–3) has defined three ways to attempt to evaluate the quality of care as follows:

> *Appraisal of structure* involves the evaluation of the settings and instrumentalities available and used for the provision of care. While including the physical aspects of facilities and equipment, structural appraisal goes far beyond to encompass the characteristics of the administrative organization and qualifications of health professionals. The term *structure* as used here also signifies the properties and resources used to provide care and the manner in which they are organized.
>
> Two major assumptions are made when structure is taken as an indicator of quality: first, that better care is more likely to be provided when better qualified staff, improved physical facilities and sounder fiscal and administrative organization are employed. Second, that we know enough to identify what is "good" in terms of staff, physical structure and formal organization. That staff qualifications, physical structure and formal organization are not equaled with quality must be emphasized. It is only expected that there be a relationship between these structural elements and the quality of care, so that given good structural properties, good care is more likely (though not certain to occur). Devices like licensure, certification of facilities, and accreditation are based largely on these assumptions. . . . *assessment of process* as the evaluation of activities of physicians and other health professionals in the management of patients. The criterion generally used is the degree to which management of patients conforms with the standards and expectations of the respective professions. . . . When evaluation of process is the basis for judgments concerning quality . . . there is the explicit or implicit assumption that particular elements and aspects of care are known to be specifically related to successful or unsuccessful outcomes or end results.
>
> *Assessment of outcomes* is the evaluation of end results in terms of health and satisfaction. That this evaluation in many ways provides the final evidence of whether care has been good, bad, or indifferent is so because of broad fundamental social and professional agreement on what results are brought about, at least to a significant degree, by good care.

The age-old question of what constitutes good nursing care continues to plague national experts and authorities ("Measures of Quality Nursing

Care?" 1976). Dr. Donabedian (1969, p. 186) more recently stated that the "seductive simplicity of the structure-process-outcome formulation can readily lead to its abuse. . . . We need to use all three simultaneously. . . . A thorough grasp of these relationships is the only valid basis for corrective or preventive action to safeguard quality." Williamson (1971) has stressed the need to relate outcome and process assessments. Thus, it can be seen that the three important components of structure, process, and outcome are essential to quality control and should be used in concert.

NURSING AUDIT—A MANAGEMENT TOOL

The nursing audit approach to ascertaining the quality of nursing has been used for more than 20 years. During that time, the nursing audit has taken on a variety of forms depending on many factors, including institutional setting. Still, the nursing audit continues to be one of the primary management tools in nursing to review the quality of nursing care delivered. Many of the nursing audits have been based on the model suggested by Phaneuf (1964, 1966, 1968, 1969, 1972), which is process oriented using the work of Lesnik and Anderson (1955) as a foundation. Support for the concept of reviewing records as a valuable source of information in evaluating the proficiency of nursing care has been suggested by many individuals (Fessel & Van Brant, 1972; Blumberg & Drew, 1963). Expert observation of nursing performance was suggested.

Carl Rinker, a field representative of the Joint Commission on Accreditation of Hospitals (JCAH) recently stated that the "nursing audit is the surveillance and evaluation of the condition in which the patient left the hospital. We investigate the plan for the care of that patient. It's the heart of the reason the patient was in the hospital in the first place—to obtain a desired condition at the time of discharge" (Ellis, 1976, p. 76). The JCAH approach to the nursing audit, which was recently developed, uses patient outcomes in relation to projected outcome criteria as predicated by medical and nursing diagnosis (PEP, 1974). The exception principle provides the focus of the audit review. Trends of practice deviation, when identified, constitute the basis for process audits and act as indicators for corrective management action.

Earlier standards developed by JCAH for quality of nursing care considered primarily the structure approach more so than process or outcome criteria. These standards tended to be somewhat subjective in nature. However, the current thrust of the inclusion of patient-outcome criteria as a basis for identifying deviation trends in practice and possible reluctant process review provides a much more comprehensive and, perhaps, more objective focus for the accreditation process.

PROFESSIONAL STANDARDS REVIEW ORGANIZATIONS
(PSRO)

"A major force in stimulating nurses' present concern with accountability has been quality assurance programs in health care mandated in Public Law 92-603 [1972 amendments to the Social Security Act] which provided for the creation of PSROs" (Ellis, 1975, p. 169).

The PSRO concept was initially conceived as establishing a professional review mechanism operating on a systematic basis to determine the necessity and appropriateness of medical care services as well as assuring the quality of care provided. The purpose of the PSRO as defined in Section 1151 of P.L. 92-603 states that:

> In order to promote the effective, efficient, and economical delivery of health care services of proper quality for which payment may be made (in whole or part) under this Act and in recognition of the interests of patients, the public, practitioners, and providers in improved health care services, it is the purpose of this part to assure, through the application of suitable procedures of professional standards review, that the services for which payment may be made under the Social Security Act will conform to appropriate professional standards for the provision of health care and that payment for such services will be made

> 1 only when, and to the extent, medically necessary, as determined in the exercise of reasonable limits of professional discretion; and
> 2 in the case of services provided by a hospital or other health care facility on an inpatient basis, only when and for such period as such services cannot, consistent with professionally recognized health care standards, effectively be provided on an outpatient basis or more economically in an inpatient health care facility of a different type, as determined in the exercise of reasonable limits of professional discretion.

The primary thrust of the PSRO was to review physician-delivered patient care. However, as the final legislation appeared, it presented certain problems. Reporting in the *New England Journal of Medicine,* Ginzberg (1975, p. 366) states that in the PSRO legislation, "The term quality is used when reference is made to so many discrete aspects of health care, such as access, availability, appropriateness, cost effectiveness, that it is impossible to arrive at a definition of 'quality' that is acceptable as well as useful. Nevertheless, the passage of the PSRO legislation demanded that one address quality, even without agreement about its meaning . . . " The concepts as suggested in the legislation tended to act as countervailing forces in many cases, so that much clarification will be needed before effective implementation can be secured.

In addition to including many discrete aspects of health care, the legislation also provided for the inclusion of nonphysician health-care practitioners. Mechanisms were implemented whereby nonphysician practitioners would have input into the process. The specification of this nonphysician input was outlined in the U.S. (HEW) *PSRO Program Manual* (1974, pp. 31–33) as follows:

> **1** Development of an ongoing modification of norms, criteria, and standards for their areas of practice.
>
> **2** Development of review mechanisms to be used for peer assessment of the performance on nonphysician health care practitioners.
>
> **3** Conduct of health care review of nonphysician health care practitioners by their peers.
>
> **4** Where care is provided jointly by physicians and nonphysician health care practitioners, there should be joint development of criteria and joint assessment of care by peer physician and nonphysician practitioners.
>
> **5** Where appropriate, participation of both physician and nonphysician health care practitioners in review committee activities.
>
> **6** Working with established continuing education programs to assure utilization of results of review in educational efforts.

The apparent lack of specificity with regard to a definitional basis for quality by the PSRO legislation did not deter the American Nurses' Association (1973) from finalizing and publishing standards. This approach was totally fitting with the basic philosophy and orientation of the ANA which has recognized for years nurses' responsibility for monitoring the quality of nursing care and services delivered, as well as the release of standards for practice in major clinical areas as a professional responsibility to society (American Nurses' Association, 1973).

Ellis (1975, p. 178) forecasts the future role of nursing in the PSRO program when she states that

> involvement . . . may include developing criteria justifying admission to hospitals or other types of facilities. Where level-of-care criteria will be needed to justify admission, nurses should participate in the development of those criteria. As methodologies for review in these settings are developed, there will be concern for the quality of nursing care provided. . . . PSRO is forcing nurses to be more specific and analytical about their area of practice. . . . Nurses will soon be able to state where and how nursing care makes a difference in what happens with the patient.

Thus, it is quite evident that the PSRO program has already had a significant impact on nursing. However, these recent experiences provide only the tip of the iceberg in terms of what we in nursing can expect from future developments of the PSRO program. It is important that the nursing profession establish the criteria by which evaluations will be made. The same approach has been suggested for the medical profession (Peer Review, 1973).

NURSING QUALITY CONTROL SYSTEM

Thus far we have examined the structure-process-outcome triad, nursing audit, and the professional standard review organization. These considerations are most helpful in attempting to ascertain information regarding quality of nursing care delivered on a unit. However, nurse-managers should develop a nursing quality control system that incorporates many of the considerations previously discussed.

This quality control system should be well planned with objectives that are compatible, complementary, and supportive of higher organizational objectives and goals. As we mentioned earlier in Chapter 3, one of the organizational goals of a hospital could be stated as follows: "The hospital shall provide quality health care to all patients (clients)." The nursing department also interprets this general goal statement and relates it in nursing terms and roles of providing quality nursing care to all patients. Consequently, these goals can be further specified for the nursing unit. An example might be as follows (modified from Durbin & Springall, 1969, p. 201):

> 1 To provide a measure which will indicate the level of quality of care and service; the degree of nursing proficiency.
> 2 To provide such measures on a continuing basis as a vital ongoing management control.
> 3 To provide feedback in order to allow the necessary managerial corrective action to assure quality of care and service.

In order for nurse-managers to be effective in securing optimal nursing-care delivery from staff, they must fully implement the goals as specified. All three goals are essential to obtain both the necessary and sufficient condition for a good quality control system.

First, nurse-managers must provide units with various measures or standards. These factors permit the basis for future comparison with actual nursing-care results to ascertain possible deviation from expectation. The initial steps in this phase of control system development include addressing the key triad—structure, process, and outcome. Following the functionalization process and the subsequent clustering of functions and activities into position descriptions, it becomes readily apparent that a staffing standard exists for each position. In each case, a thorough process of examining knowledge base, skills, and experience required is established for execution of the position. The result of this process in a generic sense determines the staffing standard for the position. Thus, a portion of the structure aspect is completed. Next, a similar process is conducted to determine the physical structure and equipment requirements. The formal organizational structure is also completed through the organizing function of management. This phase of structural standards determines the role, responsibility, and accountability and ties them together through the delegation process. The finalization of the hierarchy and completion of the span of management and control finishes the structure aspect of measurable standards.

Second, nurse-managers should set up the criteria to be used for the nursing process. To assist in the formulation of process criteria many sources may be used. Certainly the standards conceived by the American Nurses' Association (1973) can be most useful in this regard. These standards are based, to a considerable degree, on the work of Norma Lang when she was at Marquette University. Her doctoral dissertation provided much background and insight for the developers of the ANA Standards. Lang's work and the ANA Standards are based on the nursing process. The various published works of Maria Phaneuf (1964, 1966, 1968, 1969, 1972) on nursing audit processes can be most beneficial. Phaneuf's methodology is predicated on the foundational basis of the nursing process as conceived by Lesnik and Anderson. In Lesnick and Anderson's *Nursing Practice and the Law* (1955), the seven functions of professional nursing were delineated as follows:

1   Application and execution of physicians' legal orders
2   Observation of symptoms and reactions
3   Supervision of the patient
4   Supervision of others, except physicians, who contribute to the care of the patient
5   Reporting and recording
6   Application and execution of nursing procedures and techniques
7   Promotion of physical and emotional health by direction and teaching

Functions 2 through 7 are exercised through independent judgement of the professional nurse. Function 1 is, of course, dependent on the physician.

The third and final phase of the triad is the patient-outcome criterion. Basically, the outcome aspect constitutes the basis for the evaluative determination of results in terms of health and patient satisfaction. In order to establish that good measures of the quality of nursing care are properly secured, the measures must be both valid and reliable. Thus, the validity from a clinical standpoint should initially address the following questions: Did the nurse make appropriate nursing assessment and intervention decisions? Was the patient outcome up to expectations? Did other evidentiary information support the contention that optimal nursing care was, in fact, delivered to the patient? (PEP, 1974, Audit 4, modified) Nurse-managers must ascertain that the proposed measures are reliable. With this aspect managers should examine how the measures were developed and implemented. These factors relate to how the quality was defined, to the frequency of occurrence that measured state should exist, and if the measurement implementation was accomplished in an effective manner (PEP, 1974). Once nurse-managers are satisfied that the measures are valid and reliable, then it is reasonable to consider their use for managerial decision making in the nursing quality control system. The measures usually used are developed by a hospital nursing audit committee.

Next, with the establishment of measures that indicate the level of quality of care and service, nurse-managers should determine the various methods to be used in securing information to measure actual practice against criteria. Obviously, a multisource information collection system would be needed. Initially, one source of information comes from nurse-managers' observation of staff in their practice delivery. Visual observation of patient behavior and progress can also be possible indications of quality. Similarly, information secured directly from the family can provide insights into situations that might signal potential problems in patient-care delivery. However, as previously covered under Group Dynamics in Nursing (Chapter 18), the complexity of the nursing environment precludes this approach from being the primary source of information.

For this reason, nurse-managers must be astutely attuned to the information provided by the postshift report conference compared to the preshift report conference. Perceived changes in patient conditions should be explored to ascertain deviations from expectations as delineated in nursing-care plans. Identified deviations must be established as either controllable or uncontrollable. If the apparent deviation is related to nursing staff problems, then appropriate modification of future patient-care delivery should be secured through staff consultation and counseling. If the deviation is a result of essentially uncontrollable conditions of the patient, appropriate changes in the nursing-care plan should be made to meet these changed conditions. The report conference is an excellent daily method of information exchange whereby nurse-managers can obtain insight into the quality of care being delivered as a byproduct of the status reports of patient conditions and their changes during the shift. Thus, nurse-managers have the responsibility during the report conference of reviewing information from staff, identifying deviations, and taking appropriate managerial action to assist in the daily control of quality being delivered to patients. Other conferences such as case and content conferences provide additional vehicles for securing optimal nursing-care quality.

As part of the total nursing department thrust to ensure that optimal quality of nursing care may become a reality, nurse-managers have the opportunity of using information secured from the formal nursing audits as conducted by a nursing audit committee. The nursing audit committee will usually select a topic for study and will establish criteria for review of practice. They will retrieve information on nursing care as indicated in records and will screen them for compliance with the written criteria. The committee then will analyze the information to determine if in the case of deviation from criteria, such deviations are clinically justified or whether they appear to represent deficiencies. If deficiencies are identified, then recommendations to management are made, including possible plans for implementation. These recommendations should be viewed by nurse-managers as helpful in assisting in their quality control responsibilities. Deviations or deficiencies as identified in outcome criteria can, if generalized, lead to a review of the application of the nursing process and can result in the development of new or modified procedures to help ensure that the best quality is delivered. In some cases, this audit technique can assist in the identification of staff who may need continuing education or in extreme cases could result in staff termination. Later, the audit committee will have a followup to ensure that recommendations *have been* implemented and *are* working in an effective manner.

Thus, nurse-managers have three mechanisms that should be used in the formal quality control system to monitor activities (coordination) and secure timely feedback for managerial corrective action. These mechanisms are direct observation, conferences, and the nursing audit committee recommendations and plans. All three mechanisms are essential to any effective formal quality control system.

FINANCIAL SYSTEM/QUALITY INTERFACE

The final aspect of formal nursing control systems involves the financial system/quality interface.

As we stated in Chapter 1, Nursing will accept responsibility for the quality of nursing care to patients, some responsibility for continuity and comprehensiveness of care. As we are aware, nurses and physicians do not feel a binding drive to address the economy or cost question, since this is the purview and responsibility of the administration and the board of trustees.

However, we shall soon see that financial systems are becoming and will become more of a concern for nurse-managers. The concern will not only address efforts toward cost containment and control, but also with regard to cost and its relationship to quality. The scope of the cost question in nursing is great, primarily because personnel costs in the hospital constitute 60 to 65 percent of total operational cost, and nursing accounts for the vast majority of those costs to patients.

The American public has been expressing great concern over the rising costs of health care in this country for some time. Legislators and government agencies are responding to that concern in various ways. In the passage of P.L. 92–603, Congress mandated in Section 1155(a)(i) that:

> It shall be the duty and function of each professional standards review organization for any area to assume, at the earliest date practicable, responsibility for the review of the professional activities in such area . . . for the purpose of determining whether
>
> a   such services and items are or were medically necessary;
> b   the quality of such services meet professionally recognized standards of health care; and
> c   in case such services and items are proposed to be provided in a hospital or other health care facility on an independent basis, such services and items could, consistent with the provision of appropriate medical care, be effectively provided on an outpatient basis or more economically in an inpatient health care facility of a different type.

As written the implication is that the legislators believed that the cost of health care and the efficacy of that care provided should be reviewed on a concurrent basis. With the role of nurses expected to increase over time in this program, the impact on nursing care and related costs of nursing care could be substantial.

The Department of Health, Education and Welfare has been actively working to address questions of cost and quality. To ensure that future HEW programs adequately cover both cost and quality aspects, these concepts were included in the *Forward Plan for Health,* FY 1977–81 as goal statements for the Department's quality assurance program as follows:

> 1   A formalized approach should be developed to increase and disseminate clinical knowledge regarding the efficacy of medical practice, and to weigh the health benefits they produce against their risk and cost.
> 2   Operational quality assurance programs sponsored by the Department should be fully implemented including PSROs, UR and the quality assurance components of ESRD and HMO.
> 3   The PSRO evaluation plan should be completed and implemented.
> 4   Better methods of assessing and improving quality should be developed. Research in this area should include the development of strategies

for expanding participation in quality assurance activities beyond the confines of the health professional establishment.

5 Health professionals should be educated in quality assurance
methodologies to enable them to participate fully in quality assurance programs.

6 The Department's ability to manage quality assurance activities
must be strengthened. In particular, direction and guidance must be provided
to develop a sound bridge between operational quality assurance programs
and the HEW health agencies responsible for developing information about
health care quality.

Newmark (1976, p.81) states that "the literature reflects an impending crisis for PSROs because they face simultaneous expectations both to
improve the quality of health care in the United States and also to hold the
line or to reduce the expenditure for health-care services through the
concurrent and retrospective review of institutional and professional
patient-care services." Thus, problems do exist with the program, but
there appears to be little question that cost and quality interrelatedness
will be an integral part of our health-care system.

As previously mentioned, the role of the nurse-manager has increased with regard to responsibility for costs and budgets. Stevens (1976,
p.83) stated "Now that nurse executives have input into the budgetary
and financial systems of their organizations, the question becomes 'How
can they use those channels in the best interest of nursing and of the
patient?' Input into the budgetary process certainly gives the nurse
executive a needed opportunity to make others aware of nursing contributions to the organization and to the patient's welfare." Stevens suggests
that traditional budgets in hospitals only consider the nursing-care delivery component as a cost (or expense) to the hospital and no portion of
any financial statements and budgets recognize the contribution of nursing
care. She is recommending, basically, that nurse-managers can assist in
the allocation of resources by documenting how nursing actually generates income and by advocating charges for the level of care provided to
patients. Stevens (1976, pp.81–85) states that

> The nursing experience with quality control systems has provided prac-
> tice in assessing care and care outcomes; quality control systems could be
> adapted to the task of putting price tags on different levels of care. Thus, by
> combining quality control systems and patient classification systems, it
> should be possible to set price schedules related to both patient needs and
> standards of care . . . the nurse executive has a responsibility for exerting
> leadership in organizational decisions regarding financial priorities and dis-
> tribution of limited funds.

The more familiar nurse-managers become with budgets and financial systems, the better they can keep cost-benefit concepts central when major managerial decisions are made. The greater expertise developed by nurse-managers in working with financial systems and measuring patient outcomes, the more effective they will be in obtaining resources for nursing and the resulting improvement in quality of nursing care to patients.

SUMMARY

Formal nursing control systems consist of control processes and use of results to stimulate managerial action. Three ways can be used to attempt to evaluate the quality of nursing care: appraisal of structure, assessment of process, and assessment of outcomes. All ways of measuring quality must be used simultaneously to obtain a valid basis for corrective action.

The nursing audit is a managerial tool for ascertaining the quality of care delivered to patients. Many nursing audits are based on the Phaneuf model which used the functions of nursing identified by Lesnik and Anderson. The Phaneuf model has a process orientation. Other approaches have stressed the use of projected outcome criteria as predicated by medical and nursing diagnosis.

The professional standards review organization was established by P.L. 92–603. PSRO was conceived to have professional review mechanisms operating on a systematic basis to determine the necessity and appropriateness of medical services as well as assuring the quality of care provided. Nonphysician health-care practitioners were included under parts of this law. As a result of the PSRO, nurses are becoming more specific and analytical with regard to their areas of practice.

A nursing quality control system should be planned with objectives which are compatible, complementary, and supportive of higher organizational objectives and goals. This type of system should contain the following factors: measures to indicate the quality of care and services, information collected on a continual basis, and feedback mechanisms to permit managerial corrective action.

Sources of information for a nursing quality control system will be through direct observation, conferences (pre- and postshift, case, and content) and through a formal nursing audit process.

The final component of a formal nursing control system is the financial system/quality interface. Nurses generally have not felt that operational costs were an area of consideration. However, recent developments, primarily through the federal government, have indicated that nurse-managers will have a significant responsibility for the financial system/quality interface. It has been suggested that in this new role, nurse-managers can assist in the allocation of resources by documenting

how nursing actually generates income and by advocating charges for the
level of care provided to patients.

BIBLIOGRAPHY

Berg, H. V. "Nursing Audit and Outcome Criteria." *Nursing Clinics of North America* 4 (June 1974): 192–199.

Blumberg, M. S., and Drew, J. "Methods for assessing Nursing Care Quality." *Hospitals* 37 (November 1963): 72.

Commission for Administrative Services in Hospitals. *A Quality Control Plan for Nursing Service*. Los Angeles: The Commission, 1965.

Donabedian, Avedis. *A Guide to Medical Care Administration, Vol. II, Medical Care Appraisal—Quality and Utilization*. Washington, D.C.: American Public Health Association, 1969.

———. "Models for Organizing the Delivery of Personal Health Services and Criteria for Evaluating Them." Proceedings of the Sun Valley Forum on National Health Inc. *Milbank Memorial Fund Quarterly*, October 1973.

Durbin, Richard L., and Springall, W. Herbert. *Organization and Administration of Health Care*. St. Louis: C. V. Mosby, 1969.

Ellis, Barbara. "JCAH Field Respresentatives Report Surveying Experiences." *Hospitals,* vol. 50, no. 13 (July 1, 1976), pp. 75–76.

Ellis, Geraldine L. "PSRO's Background and Perspective." *AORN Journal,* vol. 22, no. 2 (August 1975):169–178.

Fessell, W. J., and Van Brant, E. E. "Assessing the Quality of Care from the Medical Record." *New England Journal of Medicine,* vol. 286, no. 3 (January 20, 1972):134–138.

Forward Plan for Health, FY 1977–81. U.S. Department of Health, Education and Welfare, June 1975.

Ginzberg, E. "Notes on Evaluating the Quality of Medical Care." *New England Journal of Medicine* 292 (February 13, 1975):366.

Gorham, William. "Methods for Measuring Staff Nursing Performance." *Nursing Research,* vol. 12, no. 1 (Winter 1963):4–11.

Lang, Norma. "A Model for Quality Assurance in Nursing." Unpublished doctoral dissertation, Marquette University, Milwaukee, Wisconsin, 1974.

Lesnik, M. J., and Anderson, B. E. *Nursing Practice and the Law,* 2nd ed. Philadelphia: Lippincott, 1955.

Lewis, E. P. "Editorial: PSROs and Nursing: Accountability or Countability?" *Nursing Outlook* (January 1974):21.

"Measures of Quality Nursing Care? Experts Agree Valid Approach Not Yet Found." *American Journal of Nursing* (February 1976):186.

Newmark, Gaylen L. "Can Quality Be Equated with Cost?" *Hospitals J.A.H.A.,* vol. 50, no. 7 (April 1, 1976):81–86.

Nicholls, Marion. "Quality Control in Patient Care." *American Journal of Nursing* (March 1974):456–459.

"Nursing Service Administrators: 'Times Call for Documentation'." *Hospitals,* vol. 50, no. 4 (February 16, 1976):89–91.

"Peer Review or Federal Peering?" *New England Journal of Medicine,* vol. 289, no. 19 (November 18, 1973): 1045.

THE PEP PRIMER: The JCAH Performance Evaluation Procedure for Auditing and Improving Patient Care. Chicago: Joint Commission on Accreditation of Hospitals, 1974.

Phaneuf, Maria C. "A Nursing Audit Method." *Nursing Outlook* (May 1964):42–45.

———. "The Nursing Audit for Evaluation of Patient Care." *Nursing Outlook* (June 1966):51–54.

———. "Analysis of a Nursing Audit." *Nursing Outlook* (January 1968):57–60.

———. "Quality of Care: Problems of Measurement—How One Public Agency Is Using the Nursing Audit." *American Journal of Public Health* (October 1969):1827–1832.

———. *The Nursing Audit: Profile for Excellence.* New York: Appleton-Century-Crofts, 1972.

Public Law 92–603.

Ramey, Irene G. "Setting Nursing Standards and Evaluating Care." *Journal of Nursing Administration* (May–June 1973):27–35.

Standards for Community Health Nursing Practice. Kansas City, Mo.: American Nurses' Association, 1973.

Standards of Geriatric Nursing Practice. Kansas City, Mo.: American Nurses' Association, 1973.

Standards of Maternal-Child Health Nursing Practice. Kansas City, Mo.: American Nurses' Association, 1973.

Standards of Nursing Practice. Kansas City, Mo.: American Nurses' Association, 1973.

Standards of Psychiatric-Mental Health Nursing Practice. Kansas City, Mo.; American Nurses' Association, 1973.

Stevens, Barbara J. "What Is the Executive's Role in Budgeting for Her Department?" *Hospitals,* vol. 50, no. 22 (November 16, 1976):83–86.

Taylor, J. D. "Control System Ensures Documentation of Care." *Hospitals,* vol. 50, no. 23 (December 1, 1976):83–85.

United States Department of Health, Education and Welfare, Office of Professional Standards Review. *PSRO Program Manual,* Washington, D.C.: U.S. Government Printing Office, March 1974.

Williamson, John W. "Evaluating Quality of Patient Care: A Strategy Relating Outcome and Process Assessment." *Journal of the American Medical Association* 212 (October 1971):564–569.

Zimmer, M. J. "Guidelines for Development of Outcome Criteria." *Nursing Clinics of North America* 9 (June 1974):317–321.

———. "Measuring the Outcomes of Patient Care." *Nursing Clinics of North America* 9 (June 1974):305–315.

Chapter 21

Nurse Interface with Control Systems

Once the formal nursing control systems have been designed, developed, and implemented, nurse-managers should constantly monitor the staff interface with the control system. They should watch and listen to staff for the general acceptance or rejection of various aspects of control. Many times staff will not demonstrate overt negative reactions to controls. For this reason, nurse-managers should look for covert behavior or indirect comments that may reveal underlying feelings of resistance toward controls. There is a series of symptoms that can surface from time to time, which provides nurse-managers with indicators of staff reaction to the control system. These indicators provide an opportunity for nurse-managers to be attuned early to developments that may have a substantial future impact, not only on the control system, but also for the entire system of management. Now we shall consider symptoms that will help alert nurse-managers to possible problems with control systems.

SYMPTOMS OF INTERFACE CONTROL PROBLEMS

There are symptoms that can be looked for to monitor reactions to controls. Certain symptoms are considered early warning ones because they usually occur before the appearance of more chronic and concrete indicators. One is lateness at work. Some individuals are continually late for work, and it may not constitute a major problem. However, it could be an early indicator of a feeling of unrest due to the control system. Certainly a unidimensional approach of examining lateness as a consideration is not a necessary and sufficient condition for concern. It must be coupled with other factors in the early warning system to be meaningful. The other factors to be concerned with are excessive use of sick leave and absenteeism. When an employee is using a considerable amount of sick leave, management should ascertain whether a true medical problem exists or whether sick leave is being used as an escape mechanism from work. The approach used must be discreet, because if a true medical problem exists, management does not want to convey an attitude of indifference toward that condition. Absenteeism should be looked at in the same way by nurse-managers. Certainly, managers do not want to delve into personal problems, but if the developing situation threatens to diminish a manager's effectiveness, some degree of intervention would seem necessary.

As the earlier indicators become more consistently observable and demonstrate a chronic nature, more employees usually will resign and the turnover rate of employees increases. To determine an acceptable turnover rate, it is not generally helpful to compare it with the turnover rate from nonhealth care organizations. Nurse-managers should secure turnover rates, if available, from other hospitals in the area as well as turnover rates from other units in the hospital. Certainly a unit has its own unique characteristics, so a historical rate on a month-by-month basis over the past few years would be helpful in securing any identifiable trend over time.

Concurrently through the early and later indicators there, is a series of generalized symptoms that are helpful to in this monitoring and assessment. One generalized symptom is passive resistance to management directions. This situation may be perceived by nurse-managers as a general lack of cooperation. Sometimes the resistance is not of sufficient magnitude to identify as uncooperative. However, if it continues over time and increases in magnitude, a state of directly observable uncooperative and resistive behavior will be noted by nurse-managers. This type of behavior generally necessitates that management increase the amount of follow-up to ensure that task assignments are completed and on a timely basis.

Another generalized symptom is the development of apathy by staff members. In this case, a general lack of initiative by staff exists. As we mentioned earlier, the formal organization even though well conceived and organized does not cover all possible situations that occur on a unit. This is where the informal organization and the initiative of the individual are important. The motivated staff member will fill the void of the formal structure and carry out the necessary activities to correct a developing situation. Nurse-managers can observe apathy when staff members state that they were not aware of a developing situation or they did not know what to do with it. Pleading ignorance to a situation is usually an aberration of passive resistance. In units and hospitals where position descriptions are used extensively, staff members will evade the issue by stating that the situation under discussion is not their job or is not their patient.

The generalized symptoms usually will result in a reduction of staff morale over time. As these conditions develop, nurse-managers will be increasingly involved in management intervention with staff and their roles. The amount of time spent on supervision will increase as staffs demonstrate passive resistance and apathy. The noted lack of initiative by staff members causes nurse-managers to become more directive. As the turnover of personnel increases, more and more time will be spent orienting new staff members. When the relative number of new staff increases, the amount of nurse-managers' time in supervision also increases. Consequently, nurse-managers will be expending full effort merely to keep the unit operating. The amount of time devoted to planning and organizing activities can be substantially reduced as management by crisis has become the operational hode. How can nurse-managers prevent management by crisis? How can nurse-managers provide leadership and not merely be reactive to developments on the unit? We shall now consider these questions and suggest some approaches for consideration.

ANALYSIS OF CRISIS MANAGEMENT

In order to understand how nurse-managers "allow" situations to get out of control on the unit, we will now examine the processes that lead to the crisis management. In the beginning nurse-managers worked with others in developing the necessary goals and objectives for the unit and/or department. Once these had been established, a plan was developed that considered a process of functionalization, a process of organizing including span-of-control considerations, and some systemic control processes. In a general sense, the initial planning was completed, the organizational structure was in place, and control mechanisms were in place to provide feedback of performance deviations. Personnel were hired in conformance with position standards to ensure sufficient resource capability to handle the assigned functions. Appropriate equipment and supplies were also purchased to assist staff in carrying out responsibilities. Thus, the predetermined organizational program was implemented with nurse-managers having a positive feeling that although a few problems would arise, in general everything was expected to go quite well.

Nurse-managers often observe early in a situation that performance deviations are occurring. In a traditional management sense, they apply management pressure by tightening controls and by increasing the amount of supervision to ensure compliance with established standards. As a result of these actions, staff members begin to exhibit frustration, passive resistance, and apathy. The reasons for such expressions by staff are that the increased amount of control to ascertain conformity has actually damaged their perception of self, has curtailed their work environment situation to preclude the releasing of their potential for self-actualization, and has not supported to any extent their ego needs. In situations like this, nurse-managers tend to focus on those areas of deviation from expectations and do not give positive feedback for all those activities that are in compliance with expectations. The problem encountered here is that if 90% of activities are conforming and 10% are not, the staff member will generalize the negative feedback to all activities performed. Granted, this result may not have been management's intent, but the perception of staff is felt to be real. It must be remembered that perceptions are viewed as real by staff members.

As a result of this type of action, the staff will develop various forms of resistance because they are rebelling against the imposed authority. Staff members may reach a level of performance that will barely be accepted to nurse-managers. The behavior exhibited by members can be such that performance is low; they show little drive or desire to do well, demonstrate a low degree of involvement in their work, and require much direction and supervision on the unit.

At the same time these developments are occurring with staff, nursing management higher in the organizational hierarchy may become aware that the nurse-manager is starting to let things get out of control. They may call a meeting to ascertain what has been occurring on the unit to produce such unexpected results. Top management may suggest that the nurse-manager institute appropriate systems of controls to correct the deviations and the generally observable nonproductive behavior. The nurse-manager returns to the unit feeling somewhat ego damaged and usually selects one of two approaches to this situation. The manager may, in fact, tighten even further the controls on staff or may simply withdraw from imposing further controls. Under either situation staff will continue in somewhat the same mode of behavior. Morale continues to be low, resistance is present, apathy prevails, and much supervision continues to be necessary. As can be seen, this type of corrective behavior by the nurse-manager can continue indefinitely without any foreseeable relief or improvement.Each iteration of this process does not produce the results intended by the action taken. What has happened that could have been prevented by another approach to the management of these care giving resources?

PROGNOSIS FOR THE NURSE MANAGER

What we have just observed is a very typical situation in many units throughout this country. Thinking back over the various management functions and concepts that have been discussed, what have we observed by this type of nurse manager behavior? If we examine the staff behavior that developed, it may provide insights into the management behavior that caused those types of reactions.

First, staff reacted to the concern of the nurse-manager over deviations from expectations. Negative responses from the nurse-manager provided insights to staff regarding a general negative management philosophy. The nurse-manager's emphasis on the nonconformity aspects of performance were not supportive from an individual staff member ego standpoint. Little feedback of a positive nature precluded a more balanced view of performance for the staff members. Thus, the general perception of performance by staff members through the feedback was negative. Next, the imposition of tighter controls to obtain greater conformity had the effect of curtailing individual ability to satisfy needs through the work setting. Staff members were concerned for job security because the initial feedback of performance is negative. The ego satisfaction possibilities were also thwarted. Recognition and acceptance has been precluded. Any attempt to seek self-actualization was virtually eliminated. As mentioned earlier an unsatisfied need motivates staff. However, such a state of motivation can only occur when staff members believe that the work environment is conducive to the satisfaction of those needs. When they perceive that needs will probably not be satisfied, staff members exhibit frustration and resistance in a passive sense.

The staff begins to behave apathetically. Little initiative is demonstrated and more supervision of staff is needed. Staff members exhibit a general uncooperative attitude. Staff commitment to the unit and organization is low. Why have these developments occurred? Through his or her approach to the unit environment, the nurse-manager has selected the behavior to be exhibited by staff. The behavior so selected was based on Theory X. As you will recall, under Theory X individuals dislike work, generally are not motivated, need much direction, and do not demonstrate elements of self-control. Therefore, they need a lot of supervision and direction as well as control of activities.

In the situation that we examined, the nurse-manager used a Theory-X approach to the staff. When the situation appeared to get even further out of control, more Theory X was called upon to correct the situation. This resulted in more control and more direction of the staff. A vicious cycle developed that did not lead to improvement or correction of the situation.

This type of managerial behavior can be observed in the majority of hospitals throughout the country, although evidences of change are occurring. The changes are in the direction of a Theory Y approach to managing. Recall that Theory Y is based on a positive orientation toward human nature. Under Theory Y, individuals like work, are generally self-motivated, and possess characteristics of self-direction and self-control. Thus, under Theory Y, staff would be more involved in the discussion of problems and in developing solutions to those problems. Through such involvement and open communication, the staff tends to develop a higher level of commitment to the unit and the organization. This process of sharing will greatly facilitate the level of identification with problems as well as a concomitant need to solve the identified problems by staff.

If a Theory Y approach was used by the nurse-manager, the problems would have been discussed openly with staff indicating positive accomplishments as well as areas of concern. Input would be received from staff on areas of additional effort for self-direction and self-control. Under these circumstances, staff would be sharing the concern through the involvement process and would likewise assume part of the responsibility that performance was not up to expectations. With this approach, there is little need for greater controls or more supervision, because staff members have voluntarily assumed that role to a great extent. Thus, the unit environment as established by the nurse-manager is not limiting in terms of individuals hoping to satisfy some of their individual needs. On the contrary, through the involvement process, individual egos have been enhanced by management recognition in this management decision-making process. In addition, although they have been identified with the problem, they feel that they can work to be part of the solution. Thus, the staff has some degree of control over the results and their own job security.

This type of approach does not create the great psychological distance that is likely to develop under Theory X. In contrast, the staff members tend to identify more closely with the nurse-manager. The informal organization also tends to provide greater support of the organizational effort to overcome the identified problems.

Individuals develop a feeling of self-worth whereby their ability to accomplish results is only limited by their own ability to perform. Thus, individuals have a most conducive environment for the satisfying of their needs. In this case, as individual needs are being satisfied, so the unit and organization are accomplishing their goals and objectives.

As Sherwin (1975, p. 684) so aptly states, "People just naturally want to improve things. So when one thinks about it, it is strange that 'resistance to change' is what is reported by observers of organization behavior when actually 'change' represents the best chance employees have to satisfy their psychological needs! The key to this paradox is that change is great when you are its agent: it is only bad when you are its object.''

NURSE-MANAGER and ATTITUDE

As previously mentioned, much of nurse-managers' managerial success evolves from their ability to minimize resistance effectively. The setting of the tone for discussion is of paramount importance. If nurse-managers approach the first discussion with staff with the preconception that all staff in the unit or department will resist any suggestion for change and improvement—it will most likely come true. It is rather odd but true that the nurse-managers who enter a situation convinced that people will resist usually find that given their presentation, that staff will live up to their expectations. As Lawrence (1975, p. 402) has stated,

> When resistance *does* appear, it should not be thought of as something to *overcome*. Instead, it can best be thought of as a useful red flag—a signal that something is going wrong. To use a rough analogy, signs of resistance in a social organization are useful in the same way that pain is useful to the body as a signal that some body functions are getting out of adjustment. The resistance, like the pain does not tell what is wrong but only that something is wrong. And it makes no more sense to try to overcome such resistance than it does to take a pain killer without diagnosing the bodily ailment.

Therefore, nurse-managers should not view the discussion with staff with great preconceptions concerning the perceived problem or the possible resistance level. As discussions with staff evolve, it sometimes happens that the perceived problem may, in fact, not be the real problem, or as frequently happens, the problem is correctly identified but for the wrong reasons. Thus, nurse-manager preconceptions can stifle necessary input to identify problems and/or their causes correctly.

It is important for nurse-managers to remember that the tone is set by management. Preconceptions limit valuable input. Finally, through their approach to the unit environment, nurse-managers select to a great degree the behavior to be exhibited by staff.

SUMMARY

The staff interface with the formal nursing control systems was examined. We observed that the nurse-manager should monitor the nurse-systemic interface for ascertainment of possible problems.

A series of symptoms was identified that indicates potential interface problems. Early warning indicators included tardiness, excessive use of sick leave, and absenteeism. A multidimensional approach was suggested prior to development of nurse-manager concern. Turnover was a firm indicator of problems, particularly if this rate increased over time. General symptoms that were noted included passive resistance, lack of cooperation, apathy, and a noticeable decrease in morale.

Problems that lead to a management crisis were examined. Areas of concern that led to problems included negative management approach, tightening of control measures, and focusing on deviations from expectations rather than having a more balanced approach. These problems produce the following staff behavior: low performance, little drive or desire to do well, low degree of involvement in work, need for more direction and supervision. We noted that the nurse-manager, following pressure from higher level management to control the unit, will probably tighten controls on staff even further. This process does not produce the intended results.

A prognosis was provided indicating that nurse-managers by their approach to the unit environment. The behavior selected was based on Theory X. We suggested that a Theory Y approach would have substantially effected the end results. The Theory Y approach permits a more conducive environment for the satisfaction of individual needs. We noted that when improvement is needed, it is much better to be the agent of change than the object.

Finally, the setting of tone is important for the nurse-manager and staff. Open communication through involvement should be fostered, whereas manager preconceptions should be minimized. Nurse-managers establish and to a great degree preselect the behavior to be exhibited by staff.

BIBLIOGRAPHY

Argyris, Chris. *Integrating the Individual and the Organization*. New York, 1964.

Flippo, Edwin B. *Management: A Behavioral Approach,* 2nd ed. Boston: Allyn & Bacon, 1970.

Koontz, Harold, and O'Donnell, Cyril. *Essentials of Management*. New York: McGraw-Hill, 1974.

Lawrence, Paul R. "How to Deal with Resistance to Change. *Harvard Business Review on Management*. New York: Harper & Row, 1975.

Maslow, Abraham. *Motivation and Personality*. New York: Harper, 1954.

McGregor, Douglas. *The Human Side of Enterprise*. New York: McGraw-Hill, 1960.

Sherwin, Douglas S. "Strategy for Winning Employee Commitment." *Harvard Business Review on Management*. New York: Harper & Row, 1975.

Chapter 22

Change Theory and Change Agents in Nursing

Thus far we have considered the establishment of an organization. We stated that the organization must be planned, organized, directed, and controlled. However, we cannot, and we should not, assume that our work is completed at this point. As previously mentioned, nurses operate in an environment that can be considered to be in a state of dynamic equilibrium. Thus, nursing units as a social system have their own complexity of motivational forces moving toward new equilibrium levels on a continuous basis. Levenstein (1976, p. 71) recently stated that "the convergence of a variety of factors in our social environment now makes change mandatory in our health care institutions. The rising level of expectations among formerly slighted segments of the population, altered demographic patterns that show an increase in the number of elderly citizens, social legislation that has increased government intervention in medical economics, the impact that inflation has had on hospital costs, the proliferation of unionization among hospital staff including professionals—all emphasize the need for innovation." The systemic changes that must be made are obviously not made just for the sake of change but, rather, to adjust the organization toward improvement and to meet the ever-changing needs of the environment. In other words, changes are essential for the organization to remain relevant.

NEED FOR CHANGE

There are basically two arenas for change. One is the previously mentioned need to meet the changing nature of the environmental aspects of society in general. The second arena is the internal organizational needs for improvement. Coping with change and management of the change process is an art that must be developed by the nurse-managers. McGuire (1975, p. 473) has stated that "the greatest problem we face is how to control change and how to live with it. We must learn how to direct change in a complex environment so that some of the fundamentals that we stand for are not destroyed or whittled away by political ambition playing upon consumer expectation like a fine instrument."

From an internal-operations standpoint, nurse-managers can be faced with a myriad of problems that demonstrate the need for change. Many of the problems are perceived by nurse-managers, whereas others are perceived by the staff. Nurse-managers can observe poorly motivated employees and those who continually cause trouble because of behavior in which the employee attempts to get by with a minimal amount of effort and/or work and by those who do not follow rules and who challenge authority. Staff members may express dissatisfaction about salary levels and working conditions. Some members will demonstrate a generally uncooperative attitude, whereas others will always be late for work or be absent quite often. Much of the complaints come from the work itself. Herzberg's research demonstrated that work itself was one of the basic motivators. Typical complaints from staff include: work itself does not provide a challenge (is too routine); their individuality is lost; they are unfairly treated and often ignored by management; they are given too much work so that quality is necessarily sacrificed; they cannot advance in the organization. According to Peterfreund (1976, p. 50), "strikes, grievances, tardiness, resignations, firings and so on are all visible symptoms of failure—on employees' part or on management's—to resolve people problems. They represent the end product, or at least the interim manifestation, of breakdowns in employment relationships that are costly, annoying, embarrassing, or in no one's interest. Yet, they are only the occasional evidence of a much broader, more expensive and much more debilitating behavior patterns." In general, the failure of systems to operate properly must lie with nurse-managers. They are the ones responsible and accountable for the overall effectiveness of the unit or department. Although there are numerous cases that we can all cite of the need for change, why does resistance to change exist within the system? Do people really want to maintain the status quo? Do providers of health-care services, particularly nursing personnel, want to change the system?

RESISTANCE TO CHANGE

Doody (1976, p. 51) reports that "the 1975 literature on health-care delivery . . . indicates a high degree of acceptance of the status quo by providers. To some extent, this situation is not surprising, considering the general economic climate and the uncertainty about impending legislative and regulatory proposals."

Much of the resistance that is observed in staff behavior is based upon philosophical orientations. Most staff members will complain about problems, want them corrected, but without any change that will affect them on a personal basis. This general point of view is that staff members are more comfortable and secure if the working environment and interrelationships are known. In other words, the working situation is more predictable when more things are known. If change of any form is introduced into the unit environment, the staff feels more insecure. In contrast, if staff members viewed changes as a positive force and were a part of that process, they would be instruments of the change rather than its object. In these type of situations, the insecurity level can be substantially reduced.

Staff will resist change when the change is major, such as a reorganization, which can result in a change of position, responsibility, and compensation. Thus, employees could perceive a loss in status, position, and money, in addition to the possible effects on the informal system. In the Maslow hierarchy of needs, the change process, if not properly handled, can shake the individual's entire foundation upon which previous sources of satisfaction had been secured. If the reorganization results in a potential reduction of staff, the impact can be devastating for those who are part of that reduction. In other cases, staff members will view change in terms of "what I will lose." This statement can be true but does not have to be the case. Some reorganizations can result in a realignment and expansion of responsibilities. In general, there is more concern about what might happen than about what actually happens.

Change occurs in varying amounts. As changes move along the continuum from minimal to substantial, the amount of resistance will usually increase. The role that the organization takes over time with respect to change will, to a certain extent, condition the staff toward change itself. If the organization has not introduced any kind of major change for long periods of time, staff members do not expect it as a part of daily organizational life. Hence, individuals do not generally have experience in coping with change. In the organization that introduces change on a more frequent basis, staff members are, perhaps, better conditioned to handle the coping aspects of the change. Of course, the rapid and continuous implementation of change can be overdone, such that the organization fails to demonstrate any visible stability over time. Brigid (1977, p. 85) compared change to the grief process, "Change is not easy, it can be long and painful, and it often follows the same pattern as the stages of grief (denial, anger, bargaining, acceptance) that a person in a terminal illness experiences. Change, like the grief process, may never reach the desired goal."

In addition to the differing reactions given, some staff members feel that change is an inconvenience to them and tends to preclude them from doing their jobs more effectively. This type of attitude most often occurs during the planning and initial implementation stages of change. In some situations the impact of a change is so unsettling that many staff members will actively try to resist it by attempting to strengthen the informal system of the organization. One of the most obvious actions in this regard is seen in the development of a labor union to represent the views of the staff members. This aspect will be covered in the following chapter. Given the various sources and reasons for resistance to change, how can nurse-managers approach the process of change to minimize the level of resistance? How can nurse-managers effectively handle the management of change and the management of conflict that so often occurs?

MANAGEMENT OF CHANGE

Perhaps one of nurse-managers' greatest and most challenging responsibilities is the management of change. Toffler (1970) has documented that the rate of change occurring in our environment has increased and most likely will continue to do so. In order for nurse-managers to be effective in handling change, they cannot merely allow it to happen. The introduction of change and its implementation must be planned through a series of well-thought-out strategies using a proper leadership style. The following strategies should be considered as a minimal set for the management of change.

First, the perception that change of some kind is needed sometimes emanates from a problem that nurse-managers believe is occurring on the unit or in the department. Nurse-managers should, at this point, begin to collect information regarding the apparent problem. The information should come from many sources, if possible, to prevent the bias of collecting all information from one source. Nurse-manager must be open-minded during this process, fully realizing that the perceived problem has not yet been validated and verified. It is totally possible that the initially perceived problem may be redefined, may uncover many other problems, or, in fact, may not even be the problem. Once the problem has been identified, validated, and verified, then it is reasonable to continue with the change process.

Second, nurse-managers should provide clear, concise statements of the problem to those who may be affected by future action. The early release of information by management helps prepare and condition staff that a problem has been identified and that there will be some action to correct it. With the release of information a statement should accompany the notice indicating that input will be sought in the near future from staff as part of the developmental process of establishing alternatives to alleviate the problem. This aspect of tying together the identification of the problem with the initial notification of requesting input helps reduce some tension that can arise with the conveyance of the problem to staff. During this process, it is important that nurse-managers recognize the relationship of the organizational structure and its systemic properties of employees who execute roles that cause the organization to operate. Mann (1957, p. 162) stated this condition quite eloquently, "Organizations, as systems of hierarchically ordered, interlocking roles with rights and privileges, reciprocal expectations, and shared frames of reference, contain tremendous forces for stability or change in the behavior of individuals or subgroups. Change processes need to be designed to harness these forces for creating and supporting change." The concept of staff member involvement is more germane in this type of situation. As Katz and Kahn (1966, p. 421) state, "Participation in the interpretation and analysis . . . of research findings leads to the internalization of information and beliefs. When ideas are a person's own, they are much more likely to be translated into meaningful practices." Thus, nurse-managers should actively work to incorporate staff involvement in the process of change. Such involvement by staff helps to reduce resistance and enhances understanding and commitment to change.

Third, nurse-managers must continuously monitor the impact of decision alternatives on individual members of staff. Certainly the needs of the organization constitute the primary motivational basis for the consideration of a possible change. At the same time, consideration of decision alternatives may indicate varying levels of impact on individual situations. Obviously, an alternative that would adequately meet the needs of the organization, while having a lesser effect on staff and their roles, should be given preference where possible. When the alternatives do not provide much opportunity for staffs to meet their needs, nurse-managers must secure mechanisms so that staff members can vent their frustrations. This step is necessary as previously cited in an analogy with the grief process. The frustration levels are usually expressed as anger. This level of expression must occur prior to bargaining or acceptance of change.

Fourth, in many cases nurse-managers can begin with staff members to balance the trade-offs of individual needs and those of the organization. In most situations the bargaining process has merit and value as long as organizational needs have not been greatly sacrificed for the sake of individuals. Once bargaining has been completed, the individual is more likely to reach the final stage of the process—namely, acceptance of the final proposed change. With the acceptance comes the necessary commitment by staff to implement the change and ensure that the success of the change has been substantially increased.

In order to manage this process of change properly, managers should demonstrate a changing style of leadership to meet the changing needs of the situation. Engleman (1976, p.1071) states that "There are times when effective leadership requires an autocratic style. And there are situations where a high degree of permissiveness is the best style for getting the job done. The style of leadership which produces results is not the one best way, but a changing pattern designed to fit the current needs of the organization as well as the needs of the followers." Thus, one cannot talk about the change in the environment and change in the organization, without considering change in the style of leadership to meet the changing needs of the situation. Engleman further states, "As regards both leadership and management I would stress that we are what we do—not what we say, think or hope to do. Our people hear loud and clear what we do, and this pretty much determines what happens in our organization over the long pull" (p.1043).

MANAGEMENT OF CONFLICT

Under management of change, we alluded to the trade-off of needs of the organization and needs of the individual. When attempting to effectuate change in a complex nursing environment, it can be predicted with accuracy that the staff will exhibit anger and frustration to the nurse-manager. Since we know and can expect that a conflict will most likely occur between personal and organizational objectives, an orientation and strategy for the management of conflict is necessary. Basically, the approach to be used by management should focus on the end result of securing the best use of personnel resources; consequently, the strategy must have a foundation in the understanding of human behavior. Thus, the following series of strategies are suggested to cope with the management of conflict.

First, nurse-managers should attempt to understand the impact of the proposed change from the individual staff member's standpoint. This approach does not imply that nurse-managers should accept or agree with the staff member's viewpoint, but rather attempt to understand the concern, anger, and, perhaps, hostility from his or her point of view. Certainly, individual staff members will want things from the organization that will be in their best interests. The true test for nurse-managers is to ascertain whether the staff members' views are the best for the hospital and the unit. Nurse-managers must realize during this process that differences will exist in perceptions of the situation. These identified differences are primarily due to individuals' value systems as well as their emotional states at the time. The evidences of stress exhibited by individuals are often considered by managers to be of an irrational nature. This situation can result in stress for nurse-managers who attempt to remain rational while coping with their own stress level.

Second, perhaps the best way to alleviate the stress for all parties concerned is to discuss the proposed change at length with those to be affected. The role of the nurse-manager is to listen. Through this type of counseling, by actively and earnestly listening, staff members can release the built-up inner tension that has developed into a state of conflict. This function is necessary if the staff members hope eventually to reach a level of acceptance of the change. It requires that staff members' true problems and feelings be brought out in a frank discussion of the issues. The real value of management of conflict is when nurse-managers fully recognize that conflict does exist. Without such a realization, little can be done to manage and minimize the conflict. The proper management of conflict assists nurse-managers in gaining insight into the feelings of others and in knowing that others may, in fact, see things differently than they do.

ORGANIZATION DEVELOPMENT

Thus far we have considered the need for change, the resistance to change, the management of change, and the management of conflict. Throughout this discussion a thread of a problem seems to be recurring—the problem of coping with change. The process of management of change and management of conflict addressed very real problems. However, the acceptance of change by staff does not always ensure that members are really committed. In addition, changes as proposed require a reorientation and rethinking by staff for the changes to be implemented on an effective basis. More importantly, staff should be conditioned for change whereby they and the organization can adapt better to change. One way of assisting organizational efforts and staff member efforts in coping with change is to develop an organizational development (OD) program.

According to Bennis (1969), "OD is a response to change, a complex educational strategy intended to change the beliefs, attitudes, values, and structure of organizations so that they can better adapt to new technologies, markets, and challenges, and the dizzy rate of change itself."

As organizational development became more a part of organizational life, it was apparent that OD referred to a wide range of long-term strategies for improvement of the organization (Seashore & Bowers, 1970; Golembiewski & Munzenrider, 1973). French and Bell (1971, p. 146) have defined OD as "a long-range effort to improve an organization's problem solving and renewal process, particularly through a more effective and collaborative management of organization culture—with special emphasis on the culture of formal work teams—with the assistance of a change agent or catalyst and the use of the theory and technology of applied behavioral science, including action research." Nath (1972, p. 34) reinforces this concept of scope for OD when he states that "organizational development is a process of changing behavior on a wide scale in such a way that the organization as a whole is more effective in fulfilling individual, group and organizational goals. Thus, the purpose of organization development is to change beliefs, attitudes, values and structures—in fact, the entire culture of the organization—so that the organization can better adapt to its changing environment."

It is important to distinguish between management development and organizational development. Usually the former refers to the training, education, and general development of managers to enhance their leadership effectiveness in the working environment. In organizational development, management is included as a part of the entire organizational effort to establish coping mechanisms of change. Thus, the scope is much greater under OD than MD.

Friedlander (1971, p.153) describes a framework for organizational development, which includes task characteristics, human needs and skills, and sets of relationships or structures. He states that "OD becomes a method of first helping the organization explore each of these three components separately, and second, exploring the degree of congruence among them, with a view toward maximizing the two outputs—human fulfillment and task accomplishment" (p.155). The OD program should develop or create an organizational climate of trust, communication, and openness (Williams, 1972; Drexler, Yenney & Hohman, 1977). In order to develop this atmosphere of organizational climate properly, it is essential that involvement of staff be an integral part of the OD program. Larry Hill, executive vice president of the American Hospital Association states, "It is common knowledge that commitment to change and the motivation to achieve that change does not spring up willy-nilly, full-grown, at the expressed wish of top management. The key to any successful program is staff involvement. . . . Therefore, early and extensive involvement will help to reduce rumors and resistance to change, alleviate uncertainty and anxiety, and help to gain understanding and acceptance of new programs" (Drexler, Yenney & Hohman, 1977, p.60).

The behavioral orientation of organizational development has been built on the concepts espoused by Argyris (1957), McGregor (1960) and Maslow (1954, 1965). Certainly the approach of organizational development is premised on the belief that changes in attitudes, motives, and values of individuals will greatly assist in making organizational changes. This type of program has not been used extensively in health-care settings. Other organizational settings that have instituted organizational development programs have experienced a considerable number of problems. Greiner (1972) reports that the greatest amount of concern and criticism of the OD programs has come from the practice level. In Greiner's article entitled "Six Red Flags" (1972), the following general problematical areas surfaced: the prepackaging of OD programs without prefit to organization, the placing of individual needs before organizational needs, behavior before diagnosis, examining process before analyzing tasks, and overemphasis on the informal organization and the use of the expert. From a slightly different perspective, Newton Margulies (1971) discusses "The Myth and Magic in Organization Development." He identifies the following myths of organizational development programs: myth of the OD discipline, myth of nonreasearchable variables, myth of newness, and the myth of increased effectiveness. Drawing on his experience as an organizational development consultant, Margulies states that "organizational development proponents argue that moving in the direction of OD values can lead to increases in the organization's ability to meet its goals. So far very little evidence has been presented to demonstrate that this hypothesis is true" (pp. 181–182).

Since organizational development programs are quite time-consuming and expensive, it seems reasonable, given the current level of problems, that perhaps nursing can learn from these experiences and not undertake OD programs at this time. The principal overriding concern is the emphasis on individual needs in some cases apparently at the expense of the needs of the organization. To combat this problem Luthans (1973) has proposed a new approach to the ongoing process of the management of change which he defines as "organization behavior modification." This approach has a more traditional management approach to change where management-selected goals and objectives are implemented through reinforcement and reward systems to secure favorable staff behavior. If as stated earlier, nurse-managers set the tone by which the behavior of staff is determined, then this approach may certainly have merit to effect change. At this time organizational behavior modification has not been in practice long enough to draw any substantial conclusions about its efficacy.

SUMMARY

Nurse-managers work in a dynamic equilibrium environment. Nursing units have their own complexity of motivational forces moving toward new equilibrium levels on a continuous basis. Systemic changes are made to adapt the organization toward improvement and to meet the changing needs of the environment.

The need for change comes primarily from two arenas: external environment and internal organization needs for improvement. There are many problems inside the organization that demonstrate the need for change. Perceptions for such changes come from nursing management and from staff members. The vast majority of problems are people problems.

The resistance to change is great because many health-care providers support the status quo. Staff members who constitute the primary source of grievances will resist change because it can produce a considerable amount of insecurity. In the case of a major change such as a reorganization, it can threaten the entire foundation that staff members use as sources of current satisfaction. Change has been compared to the grief process (denial, anger, bargaining, and acceptance).

Nurse-managers must develop strategies for the management of change. The introduction and implementation of change must be planned through a series of well-thought-out strategies using a proper leadership style. Strategies to manage change include identification of the real problem, provision of a clear, concise statement to staff of the problem as well as a request for future involvement; continuous monitoring of the impact of decision alternatives, bargaining with staff; and a changing style of leadership.

With a process of change comes the need for nurse-managers to manage conflict that will occur. Strategy for conflict management includes understanding the impact of change from staff standpoint and discussing frankly the proposed change with staff.

It is important for the organization and staff to be conditioned for change so that change can be better effected. One way of coping with change is to design an organizational development program. The purpose of OD is to change beliefs, attitudes, values, and structures to help the organization adapt better to a changing environment; OD has a strong behavioral orientation. Organizational development has come under considerable criticism by practitioners. A primary concern has been the extensive emphasis on individual needs over organizational needs. Organizational behavior modification approach was suggested to overcome this criticism. However, this new approach has not been sufficiently tested to draw any conclusions regarding effectiveness in coping with change.

BIBLIOGRAPHY

Argyris, Chris. *Personality and Organization*. New York: Harper & Row, 1957.

Bennis, Warren G. *Organizational Development: Its Nature, Origins and Prospects*. Reading, Mass.: Addison-Wesley, 1969.

Brigid, Sister Mary. "Nursing Reprofessionalized: A Change Process in Iowa Hospitals." *Hospitals,* vol. 15, no. 1 (January 16, 1977):81–85.

Doody, Michael F. "Will Providers Change the Systems?" *Hospitals J.A.H.A.,* vol. 50, no. 7 (April 1, 1976):51–54.

Drexler, Allan; Yenney, Sharon L.; and Hohman, Jo. "OD: Coping with Change." *Hospitals,* vol. 51, no. 1 (January 1, 1977): 58–60.

Engleman, Gene E. "Professional Self-Development of the Chief Executive." In *Chief Executive's Handbook,* John D. Glover and Gerald A. Simon. Homewood, Ill.: Dow Jones-Irwin, 1976.

French, Wendell L., and Bell, Cecil H. "A Definition and History of Organization Development: Some Comments." *Proceedings of the 31st Annual Meeting of the Academy of Management. Minneapolis, Minnesota, August 13–16, 1972, 146–153.

Friedlander, Frank. "Congruence in Organization Development." *Proceedings of the 31st Annual Meeting of the Academy of Management,* 1971, pp. 153–161.

Golembiewski, Robert T., and Munzenrider, Robert. "Persistence and Change: A Note on the Long-Term Effects of an Organization Development Program." *Academy of Management Journal,* vol. 16, no. 1 (March 1973): 149–153.

Greiner, L. E. "Six Red Flags." *Business Horizons,* vol. 15, no. 3 (June 1972): 17–24.

Katz, Daniel, and Kahn, Robert L. *The Social Psychology of Organizations*. New York: Wiley, 1966.

Levenstein, Aaron. "Effective Change Requires Change Agent." *Hospitals,* vol. 50, no. 24 (December 16, 1976): 71–74.

Luthans, F. *Organizational Behavior*. New York: McGraw-Hill, 1973.

Mann, Floyd C. "Studying and Creating Change: A Means to Understanding Social Organization." *Research in Industrial Human Relations* 17 (1957): 146–167.

Margulies, Newton. "The Myth and Magic in Organization Development." *Proceedings of the 31st Annual Meeting of the Academy of Management,* Minneapolis, Minnesota, August 13–16, 1972, pp. 177–182.

Maslow, Abraham. *Motivation and Personality*. New York: Harper, 1954.

———. *Eupsychian Management*. Homewood, Ill.: Irwin-Dorsey, 1965.

McGregor, Douglas. *The Human Side of Enterprise*. New York: McGraw-Hill, 1960.

McGuire, J. J. "Delivering People Care Amid Change." *Journal of Medical Society of New Jersey* 72 (June 1975):473.

Nath, Roghu. "New Directions in Organization Development." *Proceedings of the 32nd Annual Meeting of the Academy of Management,* 1972.

Peterfreund, Stanley. "Employees Must Have Sense of Freedom, Worth," *Hospitals,* vol. 50, no. 16 (August 16, 1976):60–62.

Seashore, Stanley E., and Bowers, David G. "Durability of Organizational Change." *American Psychologist* 25 (1970):227–233.

Toffler, Alvin. *Future Shock.* New York: Bantam Books, 1970.

Williams, Patrick M. "A Second Look at the Goals of Organization Development Programs." *Proceedings of the 32nd Annual Meeting of the Academy of Management,* 1972.

Chapter 23

Organization of the Informal Organization

In earlier chapters we considered the development of formal organizations. Then we considered the individual nurse, informal organizations, sociopolitical forces, involvement, communication, effective group dynamics, the nurse interface with controls, and change theory and change agents in nursing. All of these chapters reflect various aspects of the informal organization. We examined the basic needs of the individual, the need to be involved, how to work effectively in groups, and how to foster and effectuate change. What we have been considering were informal factors in the environment that have not been formally sanctioned by management. As previously mentioned, the informal aspects can greatly assist the individual and groups in helping to meet needs. In addition, the informal system can often enhance the effective operation of units and departments by meeting needs not identified by management. However, in some hospital settings management, including nursing management, is not responsive to the members and groups of the informal organization. This situation most often occurs when the management is autocratic and applies McGregor's Theory X on a relatively uniform and consistent basis throughout the hospital. Span of control is tight and much supervision is applied to staff by nursing management. Little staff input is received because essentially none has been sought and that which was voluntarily offered was promptly discouraged. When staff members feel that management is unresponsive to their needs and no apparent avenues are available to improve conditions, staff will seek ways to have their voices heard collectively. This process usually results in the organization of the informal organization. In other words, since the available ways and means do not exist for staff to improve their situation, an organized effort must be launched to meet these problems. The organization to be formed is a union which can represent the views of staff members formally to management. "A labor union or trade union is an organization of workers formed to promote, protect, and improve, through collective action, the social, economic and political interests of its members" (Flippo, 1966, p.449). Matlock (1972, p.41) accurately states this situation when he says, "The groups have taken up the weapons of trade unionism not only to redress the balance of power between themselves and their employers, but also to give weight to the professional judgement on the standards, performance, and quality of the services that they themselves provide, and judgement that frequently conflicts with the bureaucracies that employ them." In some hospitals these feelings were developing, and in 1974, mechanisms were formalized to make this desire to unionize a reality in hospitals. Amendments to the Taft-Hartley Law were passed in 1974 to remove the exemption of hospitals under this law and permit unionization of staff. This amendment will most likely have one of the greatest impacts on nursing-care delivery over the next 10 years with regard to the role of nurse-managers.

AMENDMENTS TO NLRA AND RECENT DEVELOPMENTS

The purpose of the National Labor Relations Act is "to encourage the use of collective bargaining as the means for establishing the wages, the hours and the working conditions for nonmanagerial and nonsupervisory employees" (Selletin, 1976, p.65).

The original National Labor Relations Act (Wagner Act) became law in 1935. It represented the first articulation of a national labor policy for the United States. The Wagner Act provided for the protection of the rights of workers to organize and, further, through an election process, to select representatives for the purpose of collective bargaining. The Labor Management Relations Act (Taft-Hartley Act) enacted in 1947 removed hospitals from coverage under the NLRA and left it so amended until 1974, when primarily through the efforts of the ANA, it was reinstated by the 1974 amendments to the NLRA. The 1974 amendments to the NLRA have effectively placed hospitals under the act and thereby "created a new challenge for hospital management by ensuring hospital employees the right to seek union representation" (Hacker, 1976, p.45).

In 1975 the National Labor Relations Board (NLRB) issued decisions that identified bargaining units in health-care delivery. Pepe and Murphy (1975) and Kane (1975) report that the following bargaining units were established by the NLRB: registered nurses, all other professionals, service and maintenance employees, business office clerical employees, and technical employees (including LPNs).

The traditional role of unions in business and industry was to seek improvements in hourly wage rates, better working hours, and improved retirement pay and hospitalization benefits. More recently, requests have been directed toward involvement in the decision-making process of management. With the increased roles of nurses in the hospital setting, a combination of traditional type requests are occurring, as well as involvement implications related to the delivery of nursing care to patients. Zimmerman (1975) reports the need for change in management's approach to the professional staff members. Others (Leininger, 1975; McClosky, 1975) state that the 1974 amendments will provide the necessary vehicle whereby the practice of nursing and patient care can be greatly influenced and controlled by the nursing profession. Cleland (1975, p.288) states quite eloquently that "only by working collectively to define and enforce standards of care will nursing be able to gain the public's recognition of the value of its service and its entitlement to greater personal reward. The negotiated contract can become a legal means to hold nursing and hospital administration accountable. Although the contract will include negotiated clauses relating to wages, hours and conditions of work, it is the factor 'conditions of work' which is of unique concern in professional collective bargaining." The success of unionization efforts by the ANA in a relatively short time were reported in a news release January 28, 1977. Thus, the impact of collective representation by nurses is beginning to be felt across the nation. What really constitutes the advantages and disadvantages of belonging to a union?

ADVANTAGES OF UNIONS

Why would a registered nurse join a union? What advantages could it provide in terms of health and welfare considerations as well as patient care? It can be categorically stated that many nurses would join a union to increase their own economic well-being. Most nurses would want to increase their own incomes. Many nurses indicate that pay scales are not equitable, and the union provides a vehicle for a more egalitarian approach.

At one time, the role of the nurse and mother in a family setting meant that the nurse's income was a second income. Today, this situation appears to be less and less true. Thus, nurses' income is either primary in nature or at least co-primary. The importance of the nurse's income has increased substantially over time.

As the role of income increased so has the role of benefits, such as hospitalization, income disability protection, and retirement programs. Unions can provide a very effective vehicle to assist employees in securing better benefits. Nurses also need improved working conditions. This need is especially great in terms of working hours, rotating shifts, and the general availability of updated equipment to use in patient treatment. Through negotiations, unions can provide means to improve these situations.

Many nurses have expressed grave concern over management's lack of understanding and unresponsiveness to requests to improve the quality of care delivered to patients. One of the primary problems relates to the lack of staff in units and departments. Staffing ratios can be established through union efforts as well as the specification of employment standards for positions. The positions are often not sufficiently defined in terms of skills required and inconsistencies exist among positions. The remuneration levels are also inconsistent. These situations cause much concern for staff members.

Nurses complain that they cannot get access to the key people in the hospital who can make changes happen, whether the changes be wages, working conditions, or general patient welfare. When the union enters the hospital environment, this problem no longer exists. Union leaders, acting on behalf of their constituent members, deal directly with top management of the hospital. When the union speaks it is speaking with the collective voice of its members in that hospital, which can be a significant number of employees. So the problem of not reaching the key people who make decisions and affect change is no longer a problem of concern. Thus, unions do have advantages in providing mechanisms to alleviate problems and concerns of employees.

DISADVANTAGES OF UNIONS

Given the number of advantages of unions, why would employees not join a union? The following factors reflect some of the reasons why there is resistance to union membership. Since nursing is a profession, it would be unprofessional to join a union. Unions exist for and usually represent non-professional employees. In addition, unions have been identified with factory workers who generally have less education than nurses. With the increased amount of formal education and concomitant status of working in a care-giving profession, such an identification with a union would be demeaning by lowering the prestige and status of nurses.

The entire educational and professional work experience of nurses is dedicated to the service of patients, with income and personal needs being secondary. If a union called a strike in the hospital, nurses could not leave their assigned patients to picket outside the hospital to get a 30-cent/hour raise. It would essentially defeat the whole purpose for which nursing was selected as a professional career.

Nursing, as a profession, has reasonably good salaries, working conditions, and prestige. The opportunities for professional growth and development are such that a union could not do much to enhance the nurses' professional standing in the community, other than interfere with direct patient care by calling strikes, work slowdowns, and so forth.

When views of the professional nurse are presented to nursing management proposing changes, management will, after due deliberation, make appropriate decisions in light of those concerned and effected by those decisions. To have a union represent the nurses' views to management would only provide another level of interference. To have nurses go directly to management is the most effective way to effect change. Why should nurses pay someone to represent them when they are perfectly capable of doing it themselves? Thus, some nurses do feel quite strongly that the unions are not an appropriate vehicle for them.

MISMANAGEMENT LEADS TO
UNIONIZATION/RECTIFICATION CONSIDERATIONS

What causes nurses to want to unionize? The answer is quite basic— mismanagement. In the vast majority of cases, nurses feel the need for unions to represent their views because management has not provided for the satisfaction of individual and group needs. What areas of mismanagement have provided the impetus for nurses and others to join unions in hospitals?

Hacker (1976, pp.45–47) has drawn on data from an attitude survey of more than 18,000 hospital employees over 10 years in identifying the following areas of mismanagement:

> "• Inequitable rotations for weekend, evening and night shift workers
> > • Irregular and substantial performance appraisal
> > • Seniority policy
> > • Lack of uniformity among hospital departments in the appreciation of personnel policies
> • Grievance procedures that favor managers and supervisors
> • Wage and salary plans that do not establish proper relationships

among various jobs and skills in the organization
- Lack of opportunities for promotion and transfer within the hospital
- Lack of opportunities for personal training and development
- Lack of leadership for ensuring the rights of employees''

These areas of mismanagement constitute major concerns for nurse-managers. Now we shall further examine some of these areas to establish some possible underlying concerns that may have fostered the identification of such areas.

It is interesting to observe that the majority of mismanagement areas reflect the failure of the formal organization to perform properly. The apparent ineffectiveness of the formal organization has resulted in the expansion and growth of the informal organization. For example, the rotation of employees should be done on a basis whereby equity concepts would dictate equal probability of assignment to various shifts. When this does not occur, employees feel cheated by having to draw a disproportionate number of less desirable shifts. Management's inability to assign personnel properly has resulted in rotations as a problem area. Irregular performance appraisals are inexcusable. The lack of timeliness should not be tolerated by employees or management. Nurses have performed their functions, but where is management to provide timely feedback? Substandard performance appraisal is more difficult to overcome. However, this problem, too, can be eliminated by top nursing management's providing training to all nurse-managers in the nursing department.

Seniority policies are a relatively easy concept to design, develop, and implement. However, "most hospitals have avoided delineating their seniority policies" (Hacker, 1976, p.45). There is no plausible explanation for this inappropriate lack of definition of policy. Certainly, unions can take great advantage of this blatant omission by hospital and nursing management. It is grossly unrealistic in the current environment to hire nurse staff members and not articulate how seniority relates to various aspects of employment, such as pay levels, amount of vacation, eligibility for hospitalization insurance and retirement benefits. This inaction by management provides the employees and the union with a viable issue on which to balance the power between employees and management.

In some hospitals, personnel policies are not uniform and where they are uniform, they are not applied on a uniform basis. Throughout the areas of mismanagement, the question of equitable treatment of personnel becomes an overriding issue and concern. It is important that the nursing department secure a clear understanding of personnel policies, and then it is incumbent on the director of nursing service to ensure that the implementation is accomplished in a uniform and equitable manner as intended by the policies. Equity is the central issue with wage and salary plans. Many times the position descriptions are not well defined, and salary levels are applied to those descriptions on an inequitable basis. As previously mentioned through the functionalization process, it is important that positions and roles be well defined. The resulting personnel standard for each position should be clear and specific. The standard wages can be applied consistently among positions in view of outside considerations, such as prevailing community rates for like positions. Proper following of this process should not provide a basis for employee concern about equity.

The final areas of mismanagement that will be considered are the lack of opportunities for promotion and transfer as well as the lack of opportunities for training and development. These two areas tend to show management's philosophical insensitivity toward the career development of unit and department staff members. Hospital and nursing management should establish a consistent policy regarding employee career development. The development of career paths for advancement will help alleviate this problem. The commitment from management to provide continuing education both inside and outside hospital will greatly assist in meeting the needs of staff members and preclude intervention by unions in this area of concern. Thus, there are many areas of mismanagement, but they can be rectified with the proper functioning of the formal organization, and the intervention of unions into the hospital and nursing environment can be precluded.

PROCESS OF COLLECTIVE BARGAINING

Jucius (1967, p.453) states that "'collective bargaining' refers to a process by which employees, on the one hand, and representatives of employees, on the other, attempt to arrive at agreements covering the conditions under which employees will contribute to and be compensated for their services." Specifically, it is a process in which representatives of a nursing labor organization and representatives of the hospital organization meet and attempt to negotiate a contract that specifies the nurse employee–hospital organization–nursing union relationship. Before the collective bargaining process can begin, it is necessary that a union be recognized as the exclusive bargaining representative of a group of employees (nurses). As Shultz and Johnson (1976, p.249) so aptly state, "Regardless of the legal climate now or in the future, negotiation from a collective bargaining point of view must begin with the recognition of a union." To receive such recognition and certification as the exclusive bargaining representative of a group of nurses, a "show-of-interest" petition must signed by 30 percent of the employees in the bargaining unit and the petition must be filed with the NLRB. If the petition meets the requirements of the NLRB, then hospital administration is advised of the petition and has the option of having a hearing prior to a formal election. In either case, an election is held under the supervision of a government agency, and if a majority of those nurses vote in favor of the union, then the union becomes so certified as the agent for the nurses.

The strength and control exhibited by the union will depend to a great extent on the form of union security that is identified in the contract. The contract usually includes many major areas (Shultz & Johnson, 1976, p.250): "preamble and purpose; term, life, duration; bargaining unit; recognition; union security; management rights; wages; reopening clause; hours of work; grievance procedure; strikes; holidays; vacations; leaves of absence; shift differentials (wages); discharge; benefits; safety." The union security aspect is the statement that reflects the extent of control the union has over its members and new employees.

The types of union security include (Flippo, 1966, pp.461– 463): restricted shop, open shop, simple recognition shop, agency shop, preferential shop, maintenance-of-membership shop, union shop, and closed shop. From the union standpoint, the latter mentioned shops represent more power and control than those mentioned earlier. The restricted shop is when management works to keep a union out of the institution—forms can be either legal or illegal. The open shop exists when neither management nor union try actively to keep a union out. The simple recognition shop occurs at the beginning of the collective bargaining process as described earlier with the certification of the union. The agency shop situation is evident when not all employees must join the union, but all employees must pay dues to the union. Preferential shops give preference to union members, and in many cases these have been in violation of the Taft-Hartley Act. In the case of maintenance of membership shops, an employee has the choice of joining or not joining the union. The union shop form greatly enhances the role of the union because the hospital can hire new employees but within a specific period of time they must join the union. The final form, a closed shop, which is illegal under Taft-Hartley, requires that an individual must be union member *prior to* being hired by the hospital.

Flippo (1966, p.469) has identified the basic phases of collective bargaining as a process:

1 The prenegotiation phase
2 The selection of negotiators
3 The strategy of bargaining
4 The tactics of bargaining and
5 The contract

We have discussed some of the components or major areas of the contract. Usually, the prenegotiation phase occurs following the signing of a contract. The hospital management will carefully document all activities required under the existing contract. Management collects data on economic conditions, salary trends, benefit trends, etc., basically attempting to anticipate all changes that may be suggested by the union with regard to contract components. In addition, management will observe the requests being made of other organizations by the union to obtain a clearer predictive picture of what to expect at time of negotiation. Most unions are well organized and will perform a similar analysis before the negotiation phase.

The selection of negotiators should be approached by both sides on a team basis. In the case of the hospital organization, it would be advisable not to have the top administrator present who may have direct authority to commit the organization. It is important that sufficient time be given to study proposals and consider alternatives. Unions will use a similar approach by indicating that certain issues should go back to the membership for review. Legal counsel attendance is advised for both sides because the resultant aspect of negotiations will be a legally binding document.

In terms of strategy and tactics, as previously defined, strategy usually refers to the overall plan to be used. Tactics represent actions taken with the overall plan or strategy. The plan should be well conceived, representing the extensive amount of work that is required to approach negotiations in an informed manner. Parameters should be established prior to negotiations on what amount of give and take is reasonable and acceptable. Experience of working with various negotiators will provide insights into their approach to negotiations. A continual reassessment of the various positions proposed must be made to ensure that the original parameters have not been exceeded in an overall sense. For this reason, it is generally recommended that an incremental approach be used whereby each clause in the contract is considered individually before going on to the next clause. When the negotiations are completed, the union will request that members vote to ratify the contract as negotiated. If a majority of members do not vote in favor of the contract as proposed, a strike may be in the offing with bargaining under strike conditions or even arbitration. If the members do support the contract by majority vote, then management signs the contract and it becomes binding on both the hospital and the union.

ADMINISTRATION OF THE CONTRACT

Once the contract has been signed, the implementation phase begins on a day-to-day basis. It must be remembered that the contract constitutes in formal terms the nature of the relationship between the hospital labor and hospital management. The actual implementation and interpretation of the intent of the contract will greatly determine the affect it will have on the management of the hospital and the rights of labor.

When the contract was under development, certain areas were identified as management prerogatives. These prerogatives indicate aspects in which management maintains control. These prerogatives usually evolve as a result of decision-making areas that have not been specifically stipulated in the formal contractual relationship. In some cases, management believes, from reading the contract, that certain areas were ones in which management prerogatives can be exercised. However, union representatives do not perceive the same interpretation from the contract. Consequently, a continual reassessment and interpretation of the contract will occur throughout the contract period. This process of interaction leads to clarification of various aspects of the contract. Thus, many of the so-called gray areas become more black and white.

During the contract period, hospital management is charged with the responsibility of the direct administration of the contract. Throughout the contract period, representatives of the union will monitor the administration by management. Any apparent deviations identified by the union will be brought to management's attention. In order to minimize the possibilities of contract deviations, hospital management should conduct training sessions with department heads, supervisors, and head nurses to help ensure the effective implementation of the contract. Without such training sessions, management can most likely expect to see a series of grievances filed due to noncompliance with contract requirements.

Jucius (1963, p.450) has defined a grievance as "any discontent or dissatisfaction, whether expressed or not and whether valid or not, arising out of anything connected with the company that an employee thinks, believes, or even 'feels', is unfair, unjust or inequitable." This definition is quite broad and certainly covers the possible ways that discontent or dissatisfaction may occur. The grievance must be based on a policy or action related to the hospital as the employer of record. Any complaint not relating to this area cannot be considered a grievance.

A grievance is processed through a grievance procedure which is usually identified in the contract. According to Flippo (1966, p.390), "The primary value of a grievance procedure is that it can assist in minimizing discontent and dissatisfaction which may have adverse effects upon co-operation and productivity." The implication for nurse-managers should be quite clear. Given the presence of a union contact as a legally binding document and the presence of a grievance mechanism, nurse-managers cannot effectively use an authoritarian approach on an arbitrary basis. The result will be grievances filed by employees. Consequently, nurse-managers will be spending a considerable amount of time in conference with union stewards and employees to attempt to alleviate aggrieved employees. Union stewards are elected by the union membership to represent their views at a department-head level in the hospital organization. Stewards are usually full-time employees of the union and are well versed in the contract conditions as well as in the situation at hand. From a management standpoint, this type of activity by nurse-managers cannot be considered an effective use of time.

The steps in a grievance procedure may be identified as follows (Flippo, 1966, p.390):

1 Conference among the aggrieved employee, the supervisor, and the union steward
2 Conference between middle management . . . and middle union leadership
3 Conference between top management and top union leadership
4 Arbitration

Not all the steps in a grievance procedure are necessary if the grievance can be resolved at a lower level. For example, if the conference among the aggrieved employee, the supervisor, and the union steward can result in satisfaction for all parties concerned, the process does not have to continue to the next step. If the issue cannot be resolved then it can continue through the process until it is submitted for arbitration. When an issue is subject to arbitration, the arbitration is conducted by an outside, independent third party who has been given authority to make a final decision on the issue. Once an arbitrator has made a decision, it is binding on all parties. If the parties do not follow the decision as given, it constitutes a contract violation and can be enforced through the judicial system. Thus, the strength of the contract can be seen in the courts of this country.

EFFECTIVE MANAGEMENT OF NONUNION PROCESSES

Hacker (1976, p.47) stated that

as hospitals prepare to face the impact of the 1974 amendments to the National Labor Relations Act, some of their priorities for the remainder of the 1970s will be to develop approaches to managing resources that will improve morale, minimize the risk of unionization, and provide better management control over their human resources. Hospitals must analyze and must attempt to formulate positive ongoing programs regarding personnel policies; personnel information systems; and preparation of managers, department heads, and supervisors to function effectively.

In order to accomplish the concepts proposed in effectively managing nonunion processes, it is essential that an ongoing management audit be performed in the hospital. To preclude the need for unions, hospital management and nurse-managers should involve staff members in the hospital decision-making processes. This involvement process means that staff would be continuously involved in providing input to management regarding their ideas, opinions, suggestions, and complaints. A venting process is therapeutic and can provide interesting insights and information to management in making more informed decisions. In addition, a periodic review of working conditions and policies that govern employees will help keep management in tune with thoughts of the staff. An example of this type of review would be in terms of personnel policies, their appropriateness, and actual implementation. The use of a management-staff committee to review policies and make recommendations can be a very viable mechanism to accomplish a relevancy test on current policies.

Certainly, nurse-managers and other managers in the hospital should be educated in the management of care-giving resources. With the advent of 1974 amendments to the NLRA, the need for much greater expertise and sophistication in the handling of care-giving resources have become a necessity. To accomplish this type of managerial expertise, hospitals must be willing and committed to devote resources to make this expertise a reality. It is only through preventive management that nurse-managers can maintain a voluntary input system rather than a system mandated by a union contract. The maintenance of a high level of management prerogatives is the only way to ensure the freedom to innovate as a manager and improve the nursing-care delivery system.

SUMMARY

The unresponsive management with no avenues available to improve conditions will lead staff to organize the informal organization. This process of "staff members wanting their voices heard" is accomplished in many cases by the formation of a union.

The 1974 amendments to the NLRA effectively removed hospitals from exemption under this law and permitted the unionization of staff. In 1975, the NLRB identified registered nurses as bargaining units. It has recently been reported that nurses are not only requesting traditional-type union demands of wages, hours, and working conditions, but are also demanding that nurses have a greater say in the practice of nursing in the hospital and in the care delivered to patients. The ANA has made significant inroads as the bargaining agents for nurses at various hospitals.

There are numerous advantages to joining a union: increased economic well-being, increased benefits, increased unit and department staffing, and direct access to hospital management.

The disadvantage of joining a union are: it is unprofessional; it is demeaning by lowering the prestige and status of nurses; if a strike occurs, nurses could not leave the patients; nursing as a profession has reasonably good salaries, benefits, and working conditions; and nurses should speak for themselves without representatives.

Mismanagement can lead to unionization. Areas of mismanagement relate to: rotation policy, performance appraisals, seniority policies, biased grievance procedures, inconsistency of wage and salary plans, lack of promotion and training opportunities, and lack of leadership. Rectification procedures can be instituted to preclude this unnecessary vulnerability of management.

For a union to represent employees, it must receive recognition and certification by the NLRB. To accomplish this recognition and certification, a "show-of-interest" petition must be filed and a vote of a majority of employees in favor of the union must be secured. Once this has occurred, collective bargaining can begin. Collective bargaining is a process involving employers and representatives of employees who try to reach agreements covering conditions under which employees will contribute to the organization and how they will be compensated for their contribution.

The strength and control exhibited by the union will depend greatly on the form of union security that is identified in the contract. The type of union security can range from little control such as a restricted shop and an open shop to much control as in the case of a union shop or a closed shop.

The basic phases of the collective bargaining process are: prenegotiation, negotiators' selection, strategies, tactics, and the contract. The administration of the contract during implementation is where the interpretation of the intent greatly determines the affect it will have on management prerogatives and the rights of labor. Hospital management is responsible for the administration of the contract, whereas the union will monitor that administration. Any discontent or dissatisfaction by employees can result in a grievance. Each contract establishes a grievance procedure for the handling of a grievance. If a grievance can be corrected to the satisfaction of all parties concerned, it can be stopped at any step in the process. The highest level to which a grievance can be processed is arbitration. In arbitration, an outside independent third party has been given authority to make the final decision. Nonadherence to an arbitrator's decision can result in court enforcement of the decision.

Hospital management, including nursing management, can preclude the intervention of a union in the hospital environment by effectively managing the nonunion process. An ongoing management audit is necessary to secure input from staff regarding opinions, attitudes, policies, and procedures. Involvement processes will enhance management decision making. It is only through preventive management approaches that nurse-managers can retain management prerogatives and have freedom to innovate and enhance the quality of care to patients.

BIBLIOGRAPHY

Cleland, V. "Taft-Hartley Amended: Implications for Nursing—The Professional Model." *American Journal of Nursing* 75 (February 1975):288.

Flippo, Edwin B. *Principles of Personnel Management*. New York: McGraw-Hill, 1966.

Hacker, R. L. "Organizational Systems for Change Offer an Alternative to Unions." *Hospitals*, vol. 50, no. 23 (December 1, 1976):45–47.

Jucius, M. J. *Personnel Management*, 6th ed. Homewood, Ill. Irwin, 1967.

Kane, T. J. "Non-profit Hospitals and the National Labor Relations Act—First Issues." *Journal of Nursing Administration* 5 (July–August 1975):15.

Leininger, M. "Taft-Hartley Amended: Implications for Nursing—Conflict and Conflict Resolution." *American Journal of Nursing* 75 (February 1975):292.

Matlock, D. R. "Goals and Trends in the Unionization of Health Professionals." *Hospital Progress* (February 1972):40–43.

McCloskey, J. C. "What Rewards Will Keep Nurses on the Job?" *American Journal of Nursing* 75 (April 1975):600.

Metzger, N. "NLRB Boards of Inquiry Have Been Used Sparingly." *Hospitals*, vol. 50, no. 13 (July 1, 1976):55–57.

Miller, R. L. "Anticipate Questions, Seek Answers for Adept Labor Relations Efforts." *Hospitals*, vol 50, no. 13 (July 1, 1976);50–54.

"Nurses' Association Top 100,000 Mark in Collective Bargaining Representation." *American Nurses' Association News* (January 28, 1977).

Pepe, S. P., and Murphy, R. L. "The NLRB Decisions on Appropriate Bargaining Units." *Hospital Progress* 56 (August 1975):43.

Sellentin, J. L. "Labor's Concern Face Management." *Hospitals*, vol. 50, no. 7 (April 1, 1976):65–67.

Shultz, Rockwell, and Johnson, Alton C. *Management of Hospitals*. New York: McGraw-Hill, 1976.

Zimmerman, A. "Taft-Hartley Amended: Implications for Nursing—The Industrial Model." *American Journal of Nursing* 75 (February 1975):284.

Part Six

The Future

The final chapter examines the concepts of differentiation and integration in organizations. These concepts are applied to hospital settings. The perceptions of attributes of organizations are expressed through the construct of organizational climate with specific attention to the hospital climate. We consider the convergence of individual needs and organizational factors and review the objectives of nurse-managers entering nursing management practice. As a final note for the future, the effective interface of management and nursing is discussed.

Chapter 24

Organization and Management of Nursing: The Convergence of Formal and Informal Systems

The functions of management have been examined from a systems point of view. These functions are planning, organizing, directing, and controlling. Traditional management theory was considered at length to provide a foundation for the management of nursing departments and units. We noted that the organizational behavior we observe and participate in as managers is not totally representative of what was initially conceived by management. The apparent incongruency is due to a myriad of behavioral influences that act to modify formal systems. The modification process that operates primarily through the informal system of departments and units can greatly determine the effectiveness of operational management. In one sense, management's ability to implement plans can be reduced or even thwarted by individuals and/or groups in the organization who are not supportive of the formal system as designed and developed. On the other hand, nursing management cannot possibly perceive or anticipate all operational problems of the unit or department. For this reason, the formal organizational system will not be totally comprehensive in anticipation of all eventualities. In this type of situation, the informal system can function quite effectively to fill the gaps of the original formal system and can help ensure the smooth operation of the unit or department. Thus, it becomes readily apparent that nurse-managers who are well grounded in traditional management theory and who understand the behavioral influences on traditional management theory can effect congruence of the formal and informal systems.

The interface of the formal and informal systems is the critical factor to accomplish the convergence of these two systems for successful nurse-managers. To examine this systemic interface properly, it is necessary that the concepts of differentiation and integration in hospitals be understood. In addition, as previously mentioned, nurse-managers, to a great extent, will determine the nature of the organizational environment. For this reason, the concept of organizational climate will be considered at length with emphasis on the hospital climate. Once these concepts of differentiation, integration, and hospital climate are reviewed, the concept of effective convergence can be achieved by nurse-managers. Now we shall consider these concepts.

DIFFERENTIATION AND INTEGRATION CONCEPTS IN ORGANIZATIONS

During the 1950s and 1960s management researchers studied the human relations movement and later the behavioral concepts as they applied to traditional management theory. The research findings generally applied to one specific type of organization or industry and, in most cases, was a piecemeal approach to organizational diagnosis and prognosis. This fragmented approach considered such aspects as styles of leadership, managerial development, and the proper type of organizational structure. Certainly the complexity of organizations and their environments precluded some researchers from examining the entire operation of organizations. "Nevertheless, the findings of these studies have often been generalized to all organizations. . . . the difficulty is that the essential organizational requirements for effective performance of one task under one set of economic and technical conditions may not be the same as those for other tasks with different circumstances" (Lawrence & Lorsch, 1969, p. 2). Lawrence and Lorsch have conducted considerable research in organization and environment and have noted that "much of the current organizational literature is directed at a fundamental question quite different from our own. Instead of seeking relationships between organizational states and processes and external environmental demands, as we are doing, most organizational research and theory has implicitly, if not explicitly, focused on *the one best way to organize all situations*" (p. 2).

Lawrence and Lorsch (1969) have directed their research toward addressing the question of management and organization of large organizations with multiple manager levels. Their areas of concern consisted of two areas: "First, as systems become larger, they differentiate into parts, and the functioning of these separate parts has to be integrated if the entire system is to be viable. . . second, an important function of any system is adaptation to what goes on in the world outside" (p. 7). As previously mentioned, the practice of medicine has experienced a proliferation of specialties over time. Likewise, nursing has followed with an extensive amount of specialization (differentiation). This differentiation was evidenced not only by functional areas but also in the scope of practice. Thus, it was not surprising to see the differentiation of critical care nursing from medical-surgical nursing. In addition, the expansion of the scope of practice was seen when staff nurses with expanded educational opportunities became clinical nurse specialists. Thus, within a nursing context, differentiation has become a reality. Clinical nurse specialists are on the unit as well as working independently in the field. These demands for change have come from the consumer environment as well as the medical environment.

Lawrence and Lorsch (1967, p. 8) state that "as organizations deal with their external environments, they become segmented into units, each of which has as its major task the problem of dealing with a part of the conditions outside the firm." So it is not surprising that "this division of labor among departments and the need for unified effort lead to a state of differentiation and integration within any organization."

The first writers in organization theory worked at a mechanistic approach of subdividing tasks and functions without adequate consideration of the possible effects on the individual. These original writers in traditional management did not fully consider the important behavioral aspects of the individual or informal group. As Lawrence and Lorsch (1969, p. 9) state, "As a consequence, they failed to see that the state of segmenting the organization into department would influence the behavior of organizational members in several ways. The members of each unit would become specialists in dealing with their particular tasks. Both because of their prior education and experience and because of the nature of their task, they would develop specialized working styles and mental processes. . . . By differentiation we mean these differences in attitude and not just the simple fact of segmentation and specialized knowledge."

To obtain indicators of differentiation, Lawrence and Lorsch have identified the following factors, not as an all inclusive set, but rather as important dimensions for consideration:

1   *Goal Orientation*—represents the difference among managers in different functional areas on their respective orientation toward particular goals.

2   *Time Orientation*—managers in different areas have different orientations toward time.

3 *Interpersonal Orientation*—represents the fact that managers in different parts of the organization will possess different orientations toward individuals, particularly colleagues.

4 *Formality of Structure*—represents measures of structures in an organization. The greater the number of managerial levels, the more formal the structure. (pp. 9–10)

These measures collectively provide a general definition for differentiation as "the difference in cognitive and emotional orientation among managers in different functional departments" (Lawrence & Lorsch, p.11). Thus, a differentiated organization has managers who are quite different from each other—that is, more differentiated according to the measures used. Likewise, if little differences existed, the organization would be less differentiated.

Lawrence and Lorsch further observed that,

> as the early organizational theorists did not recognize the consequences of the division of labor on attitudes and behavior of organization members, they failed to see that these different orientations and organizational practices would be crucially related to problems of achieving integration. Because the members of each department develop different interests and differing points of view, they often find it difficult to reach agreement on integrated programs of action. (p.11)

Thus, the more complex an organization becomes, the more it becomes differentiated. The more differentiated, the more difficult it becomes to meld these diverse factions into an effective, smooth, integrated effort. Integration then is "the quality of the state of collaboration that exists among departments that are required to achieve unit of effort by the demands of the environment" (Lawrence & Lorsch, p.11).

Baldwin (1970, p.20) states that

> the level or degree of differentiation in an organization affects the role expectation of departmental managers. The more specialized and differentiated, the more likely the manager is to place departmental objectives above those of the organization. This narrow role perception by managers can be the cause of conflict whenever joint decisions are required. In addition, managerial role occupants of specialized departments face a greater degree of departmental interdependence calling for increased levels of cooperation and coordination. This factor further accentuates the possibility of conflict within the organization.

Therefore, it is essential that for integration to occur and for the organization to demonstrate success, mechanisms must exist for the resolution of conflict.

To secure estimates of integrative activities, Lawrence and Lorsch (1969) established six dimensions to measure these activities (the first three for primary integrators and the last three for all managers):

1   Integration orientation and departmental structure
2   Influence of the integrator
3   Reward system for the integrator
4   Total level of influence
5   Influence centered at the required level
6   Modes of conflict resolution

Performance measures were established for six industries, and differentiation and integration factors were determined. Their study concluded that organizations that operated effectively in different environments were different in other respects as well. Differences existed in differentiation and in the methods used to accomplish both differentiation and integration. Therefore, different businesses require different organizational factors to be effective.

However, the businesses used in the study do not reveal the necessary factors for a hospital organization to be effective. Next, we shall consider an application of the concepts of differentiation and integration developed by Lawrence and Lorsch in hospital settings.

DIFFERENTIATION, INTEGRATION, AND PERFORMANCE IN HOSPITALS

In 1970, Eugene Baldwin completed a doctoral dissertation at the University of Florida, which applied the concepts of differentiation, integration, and performance to various hospitals in the state of Florida. His study was empirical in nature, and he gathered primary data through questionnaires, interviews, and statistical records of 14 hospitals offering a similar range of services with 210 to 500 beds. The methodology and instruments used were based on the work of Lawrence and Lorsch.

Primary differences with the Lawrence and Lorsch studies occurred in the establishment of measures of performance of the hospital as an organization. According to Baldwin (1970 (b), p. 4), "The absence of definable and generally acceptable hospital organization measures makes a normative approach to hospital performance nonfeasible. Thus, a descriptive approach to the problem of overall hospital performance evaluation is required." Since the general goals of hospitals addressed the quality of patient care, costs, and use efficiency, Baldwin considered various indices as a norm to measure against a predetermined set of criteria. Original indices included, in relation to quality, "(1) patient response, (2) opinion of medical staff, (3) quality of technical staff, (4) Joint Commission Accreditation data, (5) employee moral, (6) community attitude, and (7) the presence of quality control programs'' (Baldwin, 1970b, p.5). Indices that were reflective of effective use of resources were "(1) Hospital Administrative Service data, (2) financial position, and (3) length of patient stay" (p.5). The finalized set of indices to measure performance included: opinion of medical staff, quality of technical staff, Joint Commission of Accreditation data, Hospital Administrative Service data, and length of patient stay.

To accomplish differentiation of hospital organizations, various organizational subsystems were identified for the specific purpose of establishing and implementing the differentiation concept. Five major subsystems were determined as follows (Baldwin, 1970b, p.6):

1 Medical—doctors
2 Professional staff—nurses, radiology, laboratory technicians and other professional service employees
3 Nonprofessional staff—dieticians, housekeepers, maintenance and other auxiliary staff
4 Fiscal staff—accountants, purchasing agents, admissions, and other fiscal service employees
5 Administration—the administrators and their assistants

To measure the degree of differentiation, Baldwin used the four basic dimensions of Lawrence and Lorsch—namely, formality of structure, goal orientation, time orientation, and interpersonal orientation.

With regard to organizational differentiation, the study results indicated that differences do exist between function groups within the hospital. In terms of formality of structure, it was determined that the professional subsystem (nurses, etc.) was the most formally structured, whereas the medical doctors were the least formally structured. Thus, based on group averages from most formal to least formal, the following relationships were established:

Condition	Subsystem
Most formal	Professional (nurses, etc.)
Next most formal	Nonprofessional (dieticians, etc.)
Next least formal	Fiscal (accountants, etc.)
Least formal	Physicians

In terms of goal orientation, Baldwin (1970 (b), p.8) reports that "the physicians are the most highly oriented toward scientific knowledge of the groups and the administrative group indicates the strongest orientation toward patient welfare, as has been anticipated. However, the professional subsystem employees' strong inclination toward cost-effectiveness objectives deviated from the expected strong orientation toward patient-welfare goals." The statistical tests of significance were low in relation to these findings.

With regard to time orientation, the professional, nonprofessional and fiscal subsystems viewed time in a short-term sense. The administrators and physicians possessed a longer orientation toward time.

The measurement of interpersonal orientation, was obtained using Fiedler's "The Least Preferred Coworker" instrument (see Fiedler, 1967). The results showed that the physicians had the highest level of task orientation with the professional subsystem second highest. The administrative workers scored the highest in human relations orientation, whereas nonprofessional and fiscal groups were next highest.

Baldwin compared deviations from norm for hospitals by subsystem characteristics and then compared the deviation factors with performance of each hospital. It was concluded comparing differentiation and performance that "the hospitals ranked in the high performance category had fewer functional groups deviating from the desired organizational characteristics than did the hospitals in the medium and low performance categories. The hospitals ranked in the medium-performance groups also had less group deviation than those ranked in the low-performance category. This would indicate that organizational differentiation is a significant factor in organizational performance" (Baldwin, 1970(b), p. 13). Differentiation and performance appear to be related, but how does integration fit with performance? In their study Lawrence and Lorsch established six factors as previously mentioned that were felt to facilitate integration between departments of the organizations. Baldwin, using this approach, found that "the Spearman's rank-order correlation for the sample's quality of integration and performance rankings is significant at the .02 level." However, the strength of the relationship of performance and differentiation was much greater than the relationship of performance and integration. He concludes, "This difference in levels of significance to performance is considerable and could indicate just the opposite relationship of that proposed in the hypothesis. That is, the differentiation process is more significant to organization performance than the quality of integrative activity" (Baldwin, 1970(b), p. 21).

So it can be concluded from the work of Baldwin that differentiation in hospitals is an important activity. It would seem appropriate to consider the need to differentiate activities effectively within the nursing department. It is certainly true that nursing is currently experiencing a significant amount of mechanistic differentiation (specialization) as mentioned in a previous chapter. The key point for the nurse manager to consider is that differentiation can be accomplished in meeting patient-care needs while simultaneously minimizing the amount of integration required to ensure effective performance.

ORGANIZATIONAL CLIMATE—GENERAL CONSIDERATIONS

Thus far we have considered the concepts of integration, differentiation, and performance in hospitals. This approach provided insights into the mechanistic differentiation of activities and how these activities can affect formality of structure, goal orientation, time orientation, and interpersonal orientation among managers. Now we shall examine the concept of organizational climate. You will recall that earlier we examined the concept that nurse-managers will determine to a great extent how members of a unit or department behave. The summation of perceptions of unit and department members on the effective performance of their areas will establish the organizational climate. Thus, according to Campbell et al. (1970), organizational climate reflects a set of attributes perceived within the organization, department, or unit. The perception by staff members will constitute a view of management by staff and the resulting perception of the organization. This concept of organizational climate may be one of the most important and least understood concepts in management (Hellriegel & Slocum, 1974, p.255).

Hellriegel and Slocum (1974) reviewed the nature of organizational climate including criticism of the construct; analytical framework including analysis of measures, analysis of research, research rigor, contingencies on research; measures of organizational climate, perceptual measures of organizational climate; the research evidence, climate as an independent variable, climate as an intervening variable, climate as a dependent variable and concluded that "on a conceptual level, the organizational climate construct has relatively well-defined boundaries and suggests considerable potential for describing and understanding behavior of individuals within organizations" (p.276).

Using an organizational climate construct, Frederickson (1966) has established that organizational personnel who view the climate as rules oriented and closely supervised had more predictable performance than those personnel who worked in more loosely supervised and inconsistent climates. In addition, it was determined that more productivity can be expected of people with skills and attitudes who have greater independence of thought and action. In a later work, Frederickson (1968) found that the greater freedom permitted in the organizational structure, the greater the peer relationship and the less use of the formal structure as part of the organizational climate. These later findings would support the concepts proposed by McGregor under Theory Y.

Using organizational climate as an independent factor other researchers have found that organizational climate is related to satisfaction with
the job (Litwin & Stringer, 1968; Schneider, 1972, Pritchard & Karasick,
1973). In a similar view, Frederickson (1966) and Pritchard and Karasick
(1973) determined that a relationship existed between organizational climate and performance on the job.

Various researchers have conducted studies in various organizational
settings, but the setting of a hospital environment is much different from
most other organizations. How does the hospital setting stand in relation
to organizational climate and other factors?

HOSPITAL CLIMATE

Lyon and Ivancevich (1974) addressed the specific question of organizational climate and job satisfaction in a hospital. Much interest has been
demonstrated in the concept of organizational climate (Brayfield &
Rothe, 1951; Pace & Stern, 1958; Halpin & Croft, 1963; Forehand &
Gilmer, 1964; Litwin & Stringer, 1968; Tagiuri, 1968; Schneider, 1972).

As Lyon and Ivancevich (1974, p.636) state, "An important organization in which organizational climate has not been studied is the *hospital.*" They ask "more specifically, are research findings from
nonmedically based studies of any value to the hospital policymaker? Can
these findings be generalized to the hospital?" (p. 637).

Slocum, Susman, and Sheridan (1972) have tested the generality of
industrial based research conclusions regarding Maslow's hierarchy of
needs in a hospital setting and have determined that the concept of self-
actualization (highest level need) is very important to nurses.

In their research Lyon and Ivancevich (1974, p.639) used an eight-
dimensional Halpin and Crofts organizational climate description ques-
tionnaire (1963) as modified by Margulies (1965). The following eight
dimensions were used to measure organizational climate in a hospital:

    1 Disengagement describes a group which is "going through the mo-
tions"; a group that is "not in gear" with respect to the task at hand (10
items).

    2 Hindrance refers to perceptions by members of being burdened with
routine duties and other requirements deemed as busy work. Their work is
not being facilitated (6 items).

    3 Esprit is a morale dimension. Members perceive that they are
achieving a significant degree of task accomplishment (10 items).

    4 Intimacy refers to members' enjoyment of friendly social relation-
ships. This is a dimension of social affiliation not necessarily associated with
task accomplishment (7 items).

    5 Aloofness refers to management behavior characterized as formal
and impersonal. It describes an "emotional" distance between the manager
and his subordinates (9 items).

6 Production emphasis refers to management behavior characterized by close supervision. Management is highly directive and insensitive to communication feedback (7 items).

7 Thrust refers to management behavior characterized by efforts to "get the organization moving." This behavior is marked by attempts to motivate through example. Behavior is task oriented and viewed favorably by members (9 items).

8 Consideration refers to behavior characterized by an inclination to treat members as human beings and to do something extra for them in human terms (6 items).

The job satisfaction portion was measured through the concepts of self-actualization, esteem, and autonomy.

The results of the research revealed the following with respect to nurses: "A highly significant relationship between self-actualization and the hindrance and disengagement dimensions was found for nurses. Thus, a nurse's satisfaction with self-actualization appears to have some dependence on freedom from routine or busy work and a sense of not merely going through the motions of work" (Lyon & Ivancevich, 1974, p.641). They continue, "one priority is improving the self-actualization satisfaction of nurses, the approach should focus on reducing the burdensome duties and routine busy work, while at the same time improving the task of involvement of nurses. These two elements seem to be the best combination for improving the nurse's self-actualization" (p. 646).

Thus, it is essential to develop and maintain a congruency between the individual needs of the nurse and those of the hospital organization. The goodness of fit between the needs of the individual nurse and the organization can result in greater performance and expressed job satisfaction, than may be experienced in situations with a lesser degree of goodness of fit.

OBJECTIVES FOR NURSE-MANAGERS

In order for nurse-managers to approach self-actualization in the long run, their roles and responsibilities should be outlined for a career through the establishment of professional career objectives.

Stevens (1976, p.15) has eloquently stated the objectives that every nurse-manager should consider:

1 Have management skills and techniques second to none.

2 Adapt management techniques to the labor-intensive field of practicing nurse professionals.

3 Use management techniques to achieve goals defined by professional nursing.

4 Translate nursing and its goals to nonnurses, especially consumers, other managers, and the health professionals, including physicians.

5 Provide nursing statesmanship from her position as representative and leader of nurse practitioners.

6 Promote advancement of the nursing profession through support and utilization of nursing research.

THE FUTURE: EFFECTIVE INTERFACE OF MANAGEMENT AND NURSING

As a registered nurse working in a management position, you will have the unique opportunity of effectively blending the disciplines of nursing and management. By your expression of interest in management, you have indicated that you want the opportunity to use management approaches to improve patient care. Through the effective use of *caregiving resources* you can make this a reality of life. As Stevens (1976, p.16) so aptly states, "The nurse-administrator must learn that management is for her what a cardiac monitor is for the nurse clinician; it is only a means to another end. That end is represented in desired client health outcomes. In nursing administration, management must be subordinated to nursing goals."

Thus, the nurse-manager, through the effective use of management and nursing theory, brings collective forces together for the improvement of nursing-care delivery for the betterment of humanity.

SUMMARY

Organizational behavior is not totally representative of what was initially conceived by management. The informal system provides a myriad of behavior influences that modify formal systems. For organizations to be effective, a proper orchestration of the convergence of the formal and informal systems is necessary.

Much of the research in traditional management theory addressed specific organizations or industries and tended to produce piecemeal results. This research tried to seek out the one best way to organize all situations.

The research of Lawrence and Lorsch attempted to overcome the deficiencies of prior research by using the concepts of differentiation and integration in organization theory research. Rather than considering differentiation as merely the division of work, it was further defined as differences in attitude beyond merely the segmentation of work and specialization of knowledge. Differentiation was measured through the dimensions of goal orientation, time orientation, interpersonal orientation, and formality of structure. Differentiated organizations have managers who are quite different from each other in relation to the measures used.

The more differentiated an organization becomes, the more difficult it becomes to meld these diverse activities. To accomplish the effective, smooth operation of an organization, integration must occur. Integration is the extent of collaboration that exists among units or departments to achieve a unification of effort in response to the demands of the environment.

An application of the Lawrence and Lorsch model has been conducted by Baldwin in hospital settings. The research was empirical in nature with the gathering of data through questionnaires, interviews, and statistical records of 14 hospitals offering a similar range of services with 210 to 500 beds. The results of the research indicated that differentiation was related to performance. Integration was found to be less related to performance than was differentiation. From this research it would appear that the nurse-manager can meet patient-care needs through differentiation, while minimizing the amount of integration required to ensure effective performance.

Organizational climate, a useful construct in organizational theory research, reflects a set of attributes perceived within the organization, department, or unit. Job satisfaction and job performance have been found to be related to a positive organizational climate. Research has been conducted in a hospital climate using the organization climate construct. It was established that a nurse's satisfaction with self-actualization appears to have dependence on freedom from routine or busy work and a sense of not merely going through the motions of work. At the same time, improving the task involvement of nurses had a positive effect on perceived self-actualization. The goodness of fit of individual and organization needs can result in greater performance.

The objectives of a nurse-manager should be established to assist in self-actualization in a career sense. Drawing on the work of Stevens, we suggested several objectives. In the future, it is anticipated that an effective interface between the disciplines of management and nursing is necessary for the nurse-manager to be a viable force in the health care setting. Only through the effective use of care-giving resources can the nurse-manager harness collective forces to improve the quality of nursing care to patients.

BIBLIOGRAPHY

Baldwin, L. E. *Differentiation, Integration and Performance in Selected Florida Hospitals*. Unpublished doctoral dissertation, Gainesville, Florida: University of Florida, 1970.a

Baldwin, L. E. *Differentiation and Integration in Hospital Organizations*. Paper presented at the annual meeting of the Southern Management Association, Atlanta, Ga., November 13, 1970.b

Brayfield, A. H., and Rothe, H. F. "An Index of Job Satisfaction." *Journal of Applied Psychology* 35 (1951):307–311.

Campbell, J. P.; Dunnette, M.D.; Lawler, E.E.; and Weick, K.E., Jr. *Managerial Behavior, Performance and Effectiveness*. New York: McGraw-Hill, 1970.

Conner, E. J., and Hutt, J. C. "How Administrators Spend Their Day." *Hospitals,* vol. 41, no. 4 (February 16, 1967):41–53.

Fiedler, F. E. *A Theory of Leadership Effectiveness*. New York: McGraw-Hill, 1967.

Forehand, G., and Gilmer B. "Environmental Variations in Studies of Organizational Behavior." *Psychological Bulletin* 62 (1964):361–382.

Frederickson, N. "Some Effects of Organization Climate on Administrative Performance." Research Memorandum RM-66-21 Educational Testing Service, 1966.

———. "Administrative Performance in Relation to Organizational Climate." Paper presented at American Psychological Association Convention, San Francisco, 1968.

Halpin, A., and Croft, D. *The Organization Climate of Schools*. Chicago: University of Chicago Press, 1963.

Hellriegel, Don, and Slocum, John W., Jr. "Organizational Climate: Measures, Research and Contingencies." *Academy of Management Journal,* vol. 17, no. 2 (June 1974):255–280.

Lawrence, P. R., and Lorsch, J. W. *Organization and Environment: Managing Differentiation and Integration*. Homewood, Ill.

Litwin, G., and Stringer, R. *Motivation and Organizational Climate*. Cambridge, Mass.: Harvard University Press, 1968, 1969.

Lyon, H. L., and Ivancevich, J. M. "An Exploratory Investigation of Organizational Climate and Job Satisfaction in a Hospital." *Academy of Management Journal,* vol. 17, no. 4 (1974):635–648.

Margulies, Newton. *A Study of Organization Culture and the Self Actualizing Process*. Unpublished doctoral dissertation, University of California, 1965.

Pace, C., and Stern, G. "An Approach to the Measurement of Psychological Characteristics of College Environments." *Journal of Educational Psychology* 49 (1958):269–279.

Pritchard, R., and Karasick, B. "The Effects of Organizational Climate on Managerial Job Performance and Job Satisfaction." *Organizational Behavior and Human Performance* (1973):110–119.

Schneider, B. "Organizational Climate: Individual Preferences and Organizational Realities." *Journal of Applied Psychology* 56 (1972):211–218.

Schneider, B. "The Perceived Environment: Organizational Climate." Paper presented at Midwest Psychological Association, May 1973.a

Schneider, B. "The Perception of Organizational Climate: The Customer's View." *Journal of Applied Psychology* 57 (1973):248–256.b

Slocum, J. W., Jr.; Susman, G. I.; and Sheridan, J. E. "An Analysis of Need

Satisfaction and Job Performance Among Professional and Paraprofessional Hospital Personnel." *Nursing Research* 21 (1972):338–341.

Stevens, B. J. "Education in Nursing Administration." *American Nurses' Foundation,* vol. 11, no. 3 (October 1976):14–17.

Tagiuri, R. "The Concept of Organizational Climate." In R. Tagiuri and G. Litwin (eds.) *Organizational Climate: Explorations of a Concept,* edited by R. Tagiuri and G. Litwin. Cambridge, Mass.: Harvard University Press, 1968.

Index